THE INVISIBLE KINGDOM

THE INVISIBLE KINGDOM

Reimagining Chronic Illness

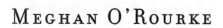

MEGHAN O'ROURKE

RIVERHEAD BOOKS

NEW YORK

2022

RIVERHEAD BOOKS
An imprint of Penguin Random House LLC
penguinrandomhouse.com

Grateful acknowledgment is made for permission to reprint the following:
Lines from John Ashbery's "A Blessing in Disguise": from *Rivers and Mountains*,
copyright © 1966, 1985, 1997, 2008 by John Ashbery. All rights reserved. Used
by arrangement with Georges Borchardt, Inc. for the Ashbery estate.
Lines from Alasdair MacIntyre's *After Virtue: A Study in Moral Theory* (2007)
are used by permission of University of Notre Dame Press.
Excerpt from *Illness as Metaphor* by Susan Sontag. Copyright © 1977, 1978 by Susan
Sontag. Reprinted by permission of Farrar, Straus and Giroux. All rights reserved.

Parts of this book have been reworked from articles that appeared in
The New Yorker, The Atlantic, and *T Magazine.*

Library of Congress Cataloging-in-Publication Data

Names: O'Rourke, Meghan, author.
Title: The invisible kingdom : reimagining chronic illness / Meghan O'Rourke.
Description: New York : Riverhead Books, 2022.
Identifiers: LCCN 2021048490 | ISBN 9781594633799 (hardcover) |
ISBN 9780593541456 (softcover) | ISBN 9780698190764 (ebook)
Subjects: LCSH: Chronic diseases.
Classification: LCC RC108 .O765 2022 |
DDC 616/.044—dc23/eng/20211117
LC record available at https://lccn.loc.gov/2021048490

International edition ISBN: 9780593541456

Printed in the United States of America
2nd Printing

BOOK DESIGN BY MEIGHAN CAVANAUGH

This book aims to provide useful information but is not intended to replace the
diagnostic expertise and medical advice of your doctor. Please consult with your
doctor before making any health decisions, particularly if you suffer from any
medical conditions that may require treatment. In a few instances, names and
identifying details of people mentioned in this book have been changed.

To all those looking for answers

Illness is the night-side of life, a more onerous citizenship. Everyone who is born holds dual citizenship, in the kingdom of the well and in the kingdom of the sick. Although we all prefer to use only the good passport, sooner or later each of us is obliged, at least for a spell, to identify ourselves as citizens of that other place.

—SUSAN SONTAG, *Illness as Metaphor*

We are never more (and sometimes less) than the co-authors of our own narratives.

—ALASDAIR MACINTYRE, *After Virtue: A Study in Moral Theory*

Contents

Part One

Obstacles

Part Two

MYSTERIES

Part Three

HEALING

Part One

OBSTACLES

INTRODUCTION

The stories we tell about illness usually have startling beginnings—the fall at the supermarket, the lump discovered in the abdomen during a routine exam, the doctor's call. Not mine. I got sick the way Hemingway says you go broke: "gradually and then suddenly."

One way to tell my story would be to say that I got ill just after college in the late 1990s, when I began experiencing daily hives, dizziness, chronic pain, and drenching night sweats, long before any doctor believed I was sick. Another way to tell my story would be to say the illness took hold in the days after my mother died on Christmas Day of 2008, when I caught a virus, a debilitating fatigue overcame me, my lymph nodes ached for months, and I slid into an exhausted fog I attributed to grief. A month later, a doctor found that I had Epstein-Barr virus. Still another way would be to say that my illness became unignorable roughly three years after my mother's death, starting in January 2012, on a windy beach by a derelict hotel in Vietnam. Jim, my partner, and I were reading by the water when I noticed a strange rash on my inner arm, seven or eight raised red bumps arranged in a circle. *It looks like Braille,* I thought. But what was it trying to tell me?

The beach was a mess that day, scattered with the skeletal, alien branches of palm trees. I was in the grips of the discomfiting loneliness that can come when wild weather presses around you. "Look at this," I said to Jim, who glanced at the angry, inflamed rash and said, "That's strange."

It was strange—stranger than I imagined at the time. I had no idea then that I was living at the edge of medical knowledge. I had been intermittently unwell since I graduated from college in 1997 and now was getting steadily worse, like a person who can't swim moving step by step into deep water. But no one knew why. At first no one even believed I *was* ill—not even I did, exactly. Trapped in a body that wasn't working, I embarked on a complicated and obsessive quest for answers. I was met by turns with cutting skepticism but also authentic concern from clinicians, friends, and colleagues. I eventually received an initial diagnosis of an autoimmune disease, but the diagnosis did not fully explain my symptoms. I tried many therapies and approaches toward healing during my search for understanding and effective treatment; in the meantime, the mysterious chronic illness I lived with got worse, not better, leaving me almost entirely unrecognizable to myself. As a child, I would wake early in the mornings with a sense of life's promise as sun drifted into my bedroom, feeling joy at what lay ahead. After I reached my sickest, I dreaded waking, because my symptoms were always worse in the morning, and because I knew the day would be full of suffering without explanation.

In the grips of a malaise I had no name for, I needed understanding. I turned to literature, science, philosophy, doctors, healers, historians, researchers, and other patients. Along the way, I became interested in the contradictions and complexities of our medical system, in the obstacles faced by patients whose illnesses are poorly understood, and in the question of what might help me live *with* illness, even if I could not overcome it. While there was no single answer, one thing stood out: above all, I wanted recognition of the reality of my experience, a sense that others *saw* it, not least because human ingenuity might then be applied to the disease that had undone me, so that others might in the future suffer less than I did.

And there are a lot of people suffering. We are all familiar with the ubiquity of long-term illnesses like heart disease and cancer, which are well-defined and viewed as unquestionably "real" (even if much remains to be learned about them). But what is less well-known is that there is also a silent epidemic of chronic illnesses that are often marginalized, contested, or even unrecognized—illnesses that include autoimmune diseases, myalgic encephalomyelitis/chronic fatigue syndrome (ME/CFS), post-treatment Lyme disease syndrome (or chronic Lyme disease, as many patients call it), dysautonomia, mast cell activation syndrome, fibromyalgia, and now, on a scale that is only beginning to be recognized, long COVID. If every age has its representative signature disease, I contend that this type of chronic illness is ours.

These illnesses are, of course, distinct from one another. But they are often characterized by dysregulation of the immune system and/or the nervous system, which are powerfully intertwined in our bodies. And some researchers suspect that there may be meaningful overlap in how these illnesses work and in the people who have them—in other words, if you have one of these illnesses, you may be more likely to have others. They are conditions that modern medicine knows surprisingly little about and that, evidence suggests, can be triggered by multiple causes, including the body's response to infections. The category is also growing in size; to take one example, autoimmune diseases are rising at what scientists call "epidemic" rates. They now affect from 24 million to 50 million people in the United States.

When I got acutely sick in 2012, such illnesses were poorly studied and rarely discussed—and often seen as manifestations of underlying mental illness. Marginalized patients who felt mysteriously unwell had to band together into activist groups to try to legitimize their suffering. A decade later, as I finish this book a year into the coronavirus pandemic, things look a bit different. Autoimmune disease is a mainstream subject. Doctors now tout the importance of the microbiome and gut health, which not long ago seemed like a fringe idea. Most dramatically, the COVID-19 pandemic has given us a keen sense of how variable the human response to infection can be, vividly dramatizing the ways that a virus or bacterium (or multiple viruses and bacteria) can collide with an individual's biology to unleash a host of perplexing aftereffects in the body, often incited by the individual's immune system. The scope of the problem of COVID-19 long haulers has begun to bring more attention to these chronic syndromes.

Even so, many people are still suffering in silence with poorly understood illnesses, and plenty of medical practitioners continue to dismiss patients like me, whose symptoms roam the body but who have what appear to be normal test results. As Susan Sontag pointedly observes in *Illness as Metaphor*, illnesses we don't understand are frequently viewed as manifestations of inner states. The less we understand about a disease or a symptom, the more we psychologize, and often stigmatize, it. Doctors once thought of multiple sclerosis as a form of hysteria. Tuberculosis (or consumption, as it was originally called) was viewed, until scientists discovered the bacterium that causes it, as a disease that afflicted romantic young souls. For decades, certain forms of cancer were thought to be a consequence of repressed emotions.

Today, we like to believe that we are rational about disease and immune to this kind of metaphorical thinking. But research shows that medicine is still riddled with such views, particularly when it comes to hard-to-identify illnesses, which are often seen as symptoms of some deeper psychological or existential problem. While advances in our understanding of mental illness constitute one of the great successes of twentieth-century medicine, patients with poorly understood illnesses confront an often reflexive categorization of their physical symptoms as mental ones—which presents a barrier to proper care and research. If medicine can't see or name the problem, it can neither study it nor treat it.

The medical uncertainty compounds patients' own uncertainty. Because my unwellness did not take the form of a disease I understood, with a clear-cut list of symptoms and a course of treatment, even I at times interpreted it as a series of signs about my very existence. Initially, the illness seemed to be a condition that signified something deeply wrong with me—illness as a kind of semaphore. Without answers, at my most desperate, I came to feel (in some unarticulated way) that if I could just tell the right story about what was happening, I could make myself better. If only I could figure out what the story was, like the child in a fantasy novel who must discover her secret name, I could become myself again.

It took years before I realized that the illness was not just my own; the silence around suffering was our society's pathology.

AND SO, THIS BOOK. It is a personal and incomplete record of my need to fathom something that neither I nor anyone else, it seemed, could understand. But it is also an attempt to synthesize what I've learned along the way, as I read, researched, and interviewed scientists, doctors, and patients. I wrote this book not only to try to explain the experience of being ill to myself, but also to help others confronted with the obstinate reality of a hard-to-identify chronic illness. (I will at times use the phrase "chronic illness" as shorthand for "poorly understood illness" or "immune-mediated illness"—that is, conditions characterized by abnormal activity of the immune system—though "chronic illness" is of course the broadest category here.)

This is a book for patients, family members, and medical professionals, as well as anyone who has faced the challenges of trying to identify an elusive medical condition. (Much of what I discuss here could be applied, say, to the experience of patients with chronic pain or migraines, or to that of patients living with cancer.) It aims to find language for a lived experience that in some ways resists description, to show how our culture tends to psychologize diseases it doesn't yet understand, and to explain how and why our medical system, for all its extraordinary capabilities, is ill-equipped to handle the steep rise in this kind of chronic illness. That system is great at providing acute care and terrible at managing the complexities of long-term care. Of course, I am not a doctor, and this account is by no means scientifically exhaustive. Rather, I hope to offer context for why these syndromes have been hard to diagnose and treat and how they challenge existing frameworks, to the extent that they are sometimes called "invisible illnesses," in the hope that it will help us revolutionize care and attitudes toward patients whose experiences have long been stigmatized. Such patients, like me, find themselves citizens of an invisible kingdom.

This account actively resists the tidiness of most illness narratives. My story does not progress in an orderly fashion, because the course of my illness did not; it circled and jumped and skipped. I got sick and better, sick and better. One self disappeared, and a new, more dependent self emerged. When I was finally diagnosed with and treated for Lyme disease, my health improved dramatically. A later diagnosis of hypermobile Ehlers-Danlos syndrome—one of a group of genetic disorders affecting the connective tissue, it is characterized by faulty collagen, hypermobile joints, pain, and fatigue—offered further explanation for my ongoing symptoms. But this is not a story of recovery or the overcoming of a disease; the focus is not on my being a survivor, or getting "better," as it is in so many illness narratives. To the degree that my quest had an object, that object turned out to be learning to live with uncertainty and incapacity. Without data or answers, I had to make room for a reality that included my near-total lack of control. I still don't have definitive answers. But gradually, peeling away uncertainty layer by layer, I arrived at what feels, to me at least, like a truth I can live with.

Indeed, this book *is* about living with, rather than eradicating or defeating, a disease: a story about letting go of the American ethos of overcoming and about confronting our mutual interdependence. My experience of being ill led me to see that our bodies may feel autonomous, but we all live in the nexus of radical interconnection. Our bodies are always in communication with other bodies: our immune system is responsive not only to collective health policies but also to the emotions and affects of others. The immune-dysregulated body, therefore, is an embodiment of our porousness to one another and of all the ways the body can be affected by personal interactions, regulation of food and chemicals, the absence of universal health care, systemic racism, poverty, trauma, and more. The coronavirus pandemic and the devastation it leaves in its wake has made this clearer than ever. But it was always true.

To have a poorly understood disease is to be brought up against every flaw in the U.S. health care system; to collide with the structural problems of a late-capitalist society that values productivity more than health; and to confront the philosophical problem of conveying an experience that lacks an accepted framework.

Even as these conditions, born of the variability of the human immune response, point to the need for a personalized approach to medical care, they also underscore the need for a stronger social safety net—and recognition of this interconnectedness. Now, with the realization that COVID-19 is further triggering epic rates of autoimmune disease and immune dysregulation, the crisis of long COVID is pushing major academic medical centers to rethink the delivery of care to such patients. Many reform-minded physicians hope that the pandemic's aftermath will lead to more change. At the same time, the formidable advocacy efforts of patient-led groups and organizations are bringing ever more attention to the problems I describe in this book. For the medical system to diagnose patients correctly, it must not dismiss their testimony.

In the end, I am one of the lucky ones, luckier than many of the other fellow sufferers I met along the way. As a highly educated white woman in the upper-income tier who lived in a major metropolitan area,

I had more resources and more privilege than many patients—and some plain old good fortune.

Another way of saying this is: I am not telling this story because I think my illness experience is extraordinary. On the contrary, what happened to me is quite common, and many people with similar conditions are far sicker than I ever was. Others receive worse care than I did. But it is the very ordinariness of my story that made it feel important to share. The words that follow are dedicated to those whom, thus far, our society has failed, and continues to fail, in the hope that change may come.

ONE

"Gradually and Then Suddenly"

I n the fall of 1997, after I graduated from college, I began experiencing what I called "electric shocks"—stabbing sensations that flickered over my legs and arms every morning, as if I were being stung by tiny bees. The shocks were so extreme that as I walked to work from my East Village basement apartment, I often had to stop and rub my legs against a parking meter; if I didn't, my muscles would twitch and my legs would jerk. My doctor couldn't figure out what was wrong—dry skin, he proposed—and eventually the shocks went away. A year later, they returned for a few months, only to stop again just when I felt I couldn't bear them any longer.

In my twenties, the shocks and other strange symptoms—bouts of vertigo, fatigue, joint pain, memory problems, night sweats, tremors— came and went. For a year, every night around two a.m., I would wake up in a sweat to find hives covering my legs, leaving me itchy and wide awake, my pajamas and sheets so wet I had to change them. Doctors prescribed a daily dose of antihistamines. There was a test that suggested lupus, and then a follow-up that showed nothing was wrong; my lab work looked fine. "The tests were all negative. It's just one of those things that will go away," a specialist told me. I remember thinking, *Don't you want to know why I have severe hives?*

In the way of women who have internalized disordered ideas about food and control, I associated my strange bouts of fatigue and discomfort with eating poorly (even though I ate a reasonably healthy diet). It was easy, in those years, to feel that a lack of dietary discipline played a role in my exhaustion, because I could tell that certain foods made me feel worse, leading me to assume responsibility for my own unwellness. I toggled between the conviction that something had to be wrong—I didn't *feel* OK—and the conviction that I was to blame, and if I just stopped eating sugar, or pizza, say, I'd be fine.

One night, I woke up suddenly from a nightmare that a man in a dirty gray sweatshirt was stabbing me. My period had started, but in addition to the cramps I had a sharp pain in my lower right abdomen. The pain grew in magnitude until, heat flushing my body, I suddenly vomited. I thought perhaps I had appendicitis, but the pain went away an hour later, just as I was preparing to go to the ER. "Everyone feels cramps," my gynecologist told me when I asked about it.

At the advice of a friend, I went to see *her* gynecologist. This doctor listened and nodded when I mentioned the stabbing pain; I felt relief at the recognition. She did an exam and ultrasound. "I think you might have endometriosis, a chronic inflammatory disease where tissue from the uterus gets out and coats the abdomen and other organs, causing pain," she said. "But it doesn't really matter unless you want to get pregnant: it can cause infertility. Later we might want to address it with surgery. For now, I'd just take ibuprofen during your period." She gave me some tissues and I wiped myself, dressed, and left, puzzled by the way my pain had been relegated to a sign that my fertility might be compromised, not a problem in its own right.

When I was twenty-four, I started waking up with a feeling that a foggy miasma filled my brain. I would go for long runs before work to clear my head, lacing up my shoes, sweating off the sleep hangover. I thought everyone felt this way, that I was just fighting a cold. But why was I so often on the verge of a cold—more than anyone else I knew? Periodically, I would start digging a little. In 2005, around the time of my twenty-ninth birthday, I was strangely enervated. I remember googling my symptoms and being struck by how much they matched those of several autoimmune diseases. I showed the results page to Jim; as the screen cast a blue light against his face, he nodded. "You are tired a lot for someone so young," he said. But then my doctors would reassure me that my lab work looked fine, and I'd return to trying to power through.

My tendency to ignore my symptoms derived in part from the fact that I grew up in a family that was largely indifferent to matters of health. As a child in Brooklyn—my parents were teachers at the school I attended—I had been raised not to think too much about my body. My parents had moved to the city from New Jersey, where they had grown up in large Irish American Catholic families. They were pragmatic and rather stoical. Like many in their baby boomer generation, they saw doctors as unquestionable experts. You didn't go to them unless you had a high fever or a bad fall or a wound that needed stitching. In that case, you got a diagnosis, you took medicine or had surgery, and you got better, more or less in that order. But if the doctor told you nothing was wrong, nothing was wrong. My parents believed in the power of Western medicine, and therefore so did I.

Ours was a family where health was not ever thought of as something to optimize or even talk about. So they took us to the doctor regularly and handed out Tylenol for fevers, but if the problem at hand was vague or seemingly minor, they tended to ignore it, telling us to buck up. As a kid, I had lots of "small things" wrong—bad allergies, muscle pain, poor digestion—which in retrospect I suspect were subtle clues about what was coming, but my parents did not pay much mind to them. I got used to being uncomfortable, and I internalized the idea that my mentioning my discomfort made me fussy—"The princess and the pea," my mother once said, in irritation, making it clear that I was demanding too much when I complained.

Still, there were moments that suggested something was not right. In July 2008, I had an early dinner with my mother—who was then on her fourth round of chemotherapy for stage 4 colorectal cancer—and my father on their patio in Connecticut. It was ninety degrees, and the sun was still up. The patio smelled of mint and basil and the air was thickly humid. I was shivering so much I put on a sweater. "You look more uncomfortable than I do," said my mother, giving me a sharp glance, her dark eyes tightening with unusual concern. "Are you OK?" I wasn't sure. When I woke up the next morning, I was exhausted and foggy headed. My mother knocked on the door, wanting to take a walk on the beach. Her black eyes were bright with the eagerness to live, and I found myself thinking that it seemed like my mother, despite undergoing chemotherapy, had more energy than I did.

All this was the backstory (not yet recognized *as* a story) to that moment in Vietnam when I found myself gazing at the angry red bumps on my wrist. *This rash means something,* I thought, trying to return to my book, as the wind whipped the palm trees and a large leaf clattered to the ground. *All these little problems—they mean something.* I stroked the bumps as if they could spell out a word that would unlock the mystery.

AT HOME IN BROOKLYN, three days after Jim and I returned from Vietnam, I developed a low fever. It was February 2012. Inside our prewar apartment the radiators hissed and clanked, sending heat through the rooms. Jim had to travel to a conference. I slept strange hours tangled in sweaty sheets. My limbs felt heavy, watery. For two more weeks, I drifted along in a flu-like malaise that I thought was protracted jet lag. At the time, to support my life as a writer and journalist, I taught in the graduate creative writing program at New York University. I had also taken a job as a visiting writer at Princeton. I was trying to start writing a new book, but it was going slowly. I couldn't seem to focus.

The jet lag did not go away.

Teaching, which I had once loved, now felt onerous. In my Monday afternoon seminar, I had trouble forming sentences. As I spoke, with my students' faces turned earnestly toward me, I felt the point of my sentences receding further and further away. I slipped out on a break for a double espresso, but the caffeine failed to clear the wooliness in my mind. I got headaches and felt dizzy when I ate; my throat was often sore. I kept reversing phrases—saying things like, "I'll meet you at the cooler water."

One morning in March, I sat down at my desk in my sunny yellow study, only to start nodding off. My body felt like a vow that had been irrevocably broken.

I wondered whether my symptoms were just the result of too much aimless internet surfing—dog videos, flash sales—and a general lack of willpower. I wondered whether I was depressed; I had experienced a mild bout of depression in college, but this was nothing like that. Open as I was to the idea, I didn't believe that I was suffering from any kind of mental illness, nor did my symptoms or recent history seem suggestive of one. My life had come together after the challenging few years following my mother's death. I had just published a memoir about her, a book I was proud of, because I felt it might help others who had suffered with feeling (as I had) that their grief was too large, too unseemly. I had been accepted into a writing residency for that summer and was excited to embark on my next book project. During my mother's illness, Jim and I had gotten divorced, our relationship strained by the devastation I felt. But now we had gotten back together and were trying to have a child. I felt lucky. I *wanted* to work; the future beckoned.

And yet I was so tired I could barely focus on my computer screen.

I called my doctor, a new internist. (My insurance had changed.) He did some blood work and phoned a few days later. "You're fine, just a little anemic," he said. Of course he did—for years, doctors had been telling me I was a little anemic, or a bit vitamin D deficient. He suggested that my fatigue was probably due to menstruation. Having menstruated since the age of thirteen without feeling on the verge of death, I found this explanation implausible and said as much. I could almost hear him shrug. "Try some iron supplements."

It's probably mono, a friend said. Maybe you're allergic to gluten, another suggested.

That weekend, on a crisp winter evening, I went to see a movie in the West Village with a group of friends. Afterward, as we headed for a drink, I began to feel shivery and shaky. I begged off. "Are you all right?" my friend Katie emailed the next day. "You seem run-down." I was sitting at my desk, looking at a photograph of myself as a teenager on a tall beachside dune playing with the family dog, a handsome black husky mix. A strong wind had turned my hair into streamers.

I couldn't remember when I had last felt that alive.

I went to an integrative doctor a friend recommended. She found that I had active infections of Epstein-Barr virus, cytomegalovirus (CMV), and parvovirus. She suggested some supplements and rest and sent me home. But I didn't feel better, even after the viruses appeared to resolve a month later. At the suggestion of a colleague, I called a doctor who specialized in women's health and made an appointment. In her office, as I described my symptoms and answered her unusually extensive questions about my family history—which included cancer, but also rheumatoid arthritis, ulcerative colitis, and thyroid conditions—the doctor (I'll call her Dr. E) said, "I can tell you now, before I even see your labs, I highly suspect that you have some kind of autoimmune disease."

The relief I experienced at hearing her say this was tremendous. Something was wrong: something, then, could be made right.

A few days later, she called to say that I had antibodies to my thyroid, a butterfly-shaped gland in the neck that regulates metabolism and energy. This meant my own immune system was attacking my thyroid, a disease known as "autoimmune thyroiditis," though people refer to this form of it as "Hashimoto's." Thyroiditis often results in abnormally low amounts of thyroid hormone, which leaves people sluggish and foggy.

I didn't worry about what the diagnosis meant; I was just happy to have one. Thyroid disease, I had read, is common and treatable. I knew people with it, and they were fine. The doctor told me to take a replacement thyroid hormone and check back in six weeks. By then, I would be feeling better. I sighed with relief. This was the way medicine worked in the modern world: tests told you what was wrong, and doctors told you how to fix it.

But six weeks later, I didn't feel better. I felt worse. My blood pressure was alarmingly low. I got headaches whenever I ate, and one day when I got out of bed I fainted. On another day, a burning pain shot up my neck; it felt as if someone were holding a candle to my skin. My friend Gina and I went to get a juice one afternoon—like me, she worked largely from home—and I got so dizzy that she had to steady me until I could sit. She looked at me as if I were really sick and said, "You need to try to get better, whatever that takes."

When I saw Dr. E again in late May, she didn't have much to say about my headaches and other symptoms, but she suggested raising my dosage of the hormone. I began to suspect that whatever was wrong with me wasn't going to be as clear-cut as a simple cold or a malfunctioning organ.

TWO

WHAT IS AN AUTOIMMUNE DISEASE?

The truth is, I had no idea what autoimmune diseases really were, even though my family had a long history with them.

Around this time, I had lunch with three of my mother's sisters—humorous, un-self-pitying Irish American women in their fifties—at my grandmother's condo on the Jersey Shore. As we ate cold cuts and drank iced tea, they told me that two of my cousins had been feeling inexplicably debilitated. "None of the doctors can figure out what it is," one said, "but I think it's thyroid related." Another aunt told us that, along with the rheumatoid arthritis she'd had for years, she, too, had recently been given a diagnosis of Hashimoto's. Both diseases were autoimmune in nature. The third aunt had ulcerative colitis and told me that a cousin did, too. "They're all connected," one explained. I'd heard the words before, but I hadn't had any understanding that the diseases might be related. This seemed like important news.

I read when I am worried, and when I got home that's what I did. I read whatever I could find about autoimmune diseases on the internet; I ordered books from the NYU library; and I downloaded papers published in medical journals. My ability to accumulate information felt like the only control I still possessed.

Within a few weeks, I had begun to understand why the Hashimoto's diagnosis might mean that something more serious—and more systemic— was going on than just a glitch in my thyroid. In a normal immune response, the body creates antibodies (Y-shaped protein molecules) and white blood cells to fight off pathogens like viruses and bacteria and then calls those cells back when the pathogen is vanquished, in order not to damage the body. Autoimmune disease occurs when, for some reason, the body creates antibodies that attack its own healthy tissue, turning on the very thing it is supposed to protect. In autoimmunity, the immune system has stopped "tolerating" the body's own tissue, failing to distinguish, as some immunologists tellingly put it, "self and non-self." ("Auto," after all, means "self.")

The question is why that self-attack happens.

It took a long time for medicine to try to answer that question. From the start, the study of autoimmunity has been characterized by uncertainty and error. When immune cells were discovered in the late nineteenth century, researchers wondered whether they might sometimes turn on us. But in 1901, the influential German immunologist Paul Ehrlich argued that autoimmunity was not possible, because the body had what he called a "horror autotoxicus," or a fear of self-poisoning. Ehrlich's theory was so fully embraced by medical science that researchers stopped exploring the subject for half a century.

In the 1950s, though, a young medical student named Noel Rose, who worked with one of Ehrlich's disciples, Ernest Witebsky, discovered thyroid autoantibodies (antibodies that attack one's own tissue) while studying the immunology of cancer. After he injected an extract of a rabbit's thyroid protein back into its thyroid, Rose found, unexpectedly, that the rabbit produced antibodies to its own tissue. Furthermore, the rabbit's lymphocytes (a kind of white blood cell) started to damage its thyroid. Rose and, eventually, Witebsky realized that they had stumbled onto something major: Ehrlich had been wrong, and the body could, in fact, be attacked by its own immune system.

In the decades since, scientists have discovered an estimated eighty to a hundred autoimmune disorders, among them lupus, multiple sclerosis, type 1 diabetes, and rheumatoid arthritis. But exact numbers are hard to come by, because researchers still do not agree on how to define an autoimmune disease. Even the term "autoimmune disease" may be imprecise: it is not known in every case whether autoimmune dysfunction is the cause of the disease or a consequence of it. Perhaps thinking of autoimmunity as the disease itself is akin to the mistake that nineteenth-century doctors made in classifying fevers as distinct diseases rather than as symptoms of diseases, as Noel Rose, who eventually became the founder of the Johns Hopkins Center for Autoimmune Research, explained to me when we spoke by phone one afternoon.

Then there is the complexity of the immune system, which I was only then beginning to grasp. The thyroid patients I followed on my social media platforms tended to be preoccupied with levels of autoantibodies, which are made in our bone marrow. But as Rose (who died in 2020) explained to me, a patient can have a low autoantibody count and still feel quite sick, or a high autoantibody count and feel fine. These uncertainties add to the shadowiness of the experience.

In some ways, autoimmune disease is as much of a medical frontier today as syphilis or tuberculosis was in the nineteenth century. One Harvard researcher told me that medical science's understanding of autoimmunity lags a decade behind its understanding of cancer (a category of disease that is itself still only partially understood). It is clear that there is a genetic component to autoimmune diseases; they tend to cluster in families, and many people end up with more than one such disease. But it is also clear that environment plays a major role: cases of autoimmune disease are rising at almost epidemic rates in affluent Western countries. Indeed, studies of twins suggest that autoimmune diseases are one third genetic and two thirds environmental, Rose told me.

Today, the Autoimmune Association (also known as AARDA) estimates that as many as 50 million Americans live with autoimmune disorders, which would make it one of the most prevalent categories of disease, ahead of cancer. A 2020 study found that incidence of antinuclear antibodies (ANA), a common biomarker of autoimmunity, has risen significantly in certain age groups since 1991, tripling in adolescents. Because, by and large, humans' genetic material hasn't changed in a generation, scientists attribute the dramatic rise to changes in environment or lifestyle, including diet and its effect on the microbiome.

Autoimmune diseases affect different groups differently, too. For reasons that are still not well understood, approximately 80 percent of autoimmune patients are women, though a handful of autoimmune diseases overwhelmingly affect men. Certain autoimmune diseases (in particular lupus) are known to affect ethnicities differently: Black women and Hispanic women are diagnosed with lupus at close to three times the rate of non-Hispanic white women and have a mortality rate that is between two and three times higher than that of white women. (And yet women of color remain underrepresented in clinical trials, as the Lupus Foundation of America pointed out to me.)

Increasingly, autoimmune diseases "represent a major disease burden—and a rapidly growing global health problem," write Warwick Anderson and Ian R. Mackay, authors of the perceptive and insightful *Intolerant Bodies: A Short History of Autoimmunity*. In 2001, the National Institute of Allergy and Infectious Diseases (NIAID) put the annual cost of autoimmune diseases at more than $100 billion. (This figure, many researchers think, vastly underestimates the true costs.) Many autoimmune diseases are associated with earlier mortality; they are the leading cause of morbidity in women, according to AARDA. Yet when I was diagnosed in 2012, few people knew what an autoimmune disease was.

My experience of feeling unwell for years before I received a diagnosis is typical. According to AARDA, it takes an average of three years (and four doctors) for a sufferer to be given a diagnosis of an autoimmune disease. One reason is that early symptoms can be intermittent and nonspecific. Then, too, a limited amount of autoimmunity itself is not necessarily considered pathological: tests often show the presence of small numbers of antibodies to your own tissues. "Autoimmune disease" is what happens when such autoantibodies produce sustained harm to your body. In some ways, the distinction between normalcy and pathology is arbitrarily defined—as well as hard to measure.

In fact, medicine still lacks good diagnostic tools for many autoimmune disorders (which is why many research institutes are at work trying to improve them). As Noel Rose told me, tests often show the presence of disease only when 80 percent of the organ under attack has been destroyed. By that time, as he put it, "The train's gone off the tracks."

Another difficulty in diagnosing autoimmune diseases is that they often present as a systemic illness, with symptoms occurring in different parts of the body, and yet our health care system is very siloed. Patients often end up consulting different specialists for different symptoms, with no one taking a big-picture look at the patient's illness, unless a primary care doctor has the time to puzzle it out. One woman I interviewed told me she was referred, over time, to a dermatologist, an endocrinologist, an immunologist, and a neurologist. She felt that each doctor she saw was just checking "his organ" off the list before telling her it wasn't the cause of her symptoms and sending her on her way. As it is, many clinicians assume that the patient, who is often a young woman, is simply one of the "worried well": people who visit doctors for reassurance that nothing is wrong with them.

I can see how my doctors might have thought such a thing about me, because I seemed on the surface to be relatively healthy—I exercised, I worked, I had a social life, and my symptoms came only in bouts. And truth be told, at first I didn't question their assessments of my health. In addition to growing up in my no-nonsense family, I had been a gymnast from a young age—and gymnastics was a sport that taught me to ignore, and overcome, pain. And so even though I fussed at times about my aches and pains, fundamentally I expected my body to heal itself. At my core, I thought my body was predictable and strong, because in many ways it *was* a tool I could train and discipline to do what I wanted. So as my symptoms accrued in my twenties, I did not understand that I might truly be sick.

My fatigue felt like a problem with *me*—something about my very being. I worked too hard, but without enough discipline; I exercised, but I ate junk food; I was sloppy where I should be ascetic. When I felt off, it was my fault, a sign of some internal weakness, a lack of moral fiber, a crack running through the integrity of my being. "It is hardly possible to take up one's residence in the kingdom of the ill unprejudiced by the lurid metaphors with which it has been landscaped," Sontag writes. Indeed: despite all my efforts to think objectively about whatever was wrong with me, I fell subject to distorting reflections. When I eventually read Sontag's words, I startled in recognition of their truth.

SINCE DR. E HAD TOLD ME it would take about six weeks for the full effects of the higher dosage of the thyroid replacement hormone to kick in, I had to wait to see if the new levels helped my symptoms. I was not feeling well enough to work, and the weeks were dragging past, so I decided I needed to do *something*. When we'd met, Dr. E had mentioned that many of her patients did better when they avoided wheat. In my reading I had learned that autoimmune conditions could be triggered by chemical exposure and by diet and that some thyroid patients are sensitive to gluten, which can exacerbate their condition. So I became hyperconscious about what I ate and what I exposed myself to. And I went online to learn more.

At one point in his memoir of living with late-stage syphilis, *In the Land of Pain,* the nineteenth-century French writer Alphonse Daudet describes staying at a sanatorium, one of those places where everyone understands what everyone else is going through. He talks about the strange pleasure of searching for the patient whose experience of illness is most like his own. Today's version of the sanatorium are internet patient groups, where one finds a vaporous world of fellow sufferers, companions in isolation and fear and frustration, as well as practitioners who have made it their life's work to understand why a segment of the population always feels unwell. I fell into the rabbit hole and emerged in another world.

On a humid day in late May, hunched over my desk, which was scattered with my medical records, I began googling "healing autoimmune disease." The world of internet illness is full of opinionated people trading tips about ideal vitamin levels, arguing about the best diets, sharing information about lab levels and helpful doctors, commiserating about fatigue. I joined a group on Facebook where I tentatively posted a question about finding a good endocrinologist. Clicking through that page and the pastel blogs, with their soothing presentations (a woman hugging a tree; a sunflower standing guard by the word "Natural"), I found people who had the same seemingly disconnected symptoms I had experienced over the years. One woman, like me, had had hives for months before an autoimmune disease was diagnosed; some had low cortisol or vitamin D and vitamin B_{12}; others had brain fog.

Most of the blog posts were carefully upbeat ("A Gluten-Free Treat for You!" and "Meditation Only Takes a Moment"), but the information was overwhelming and often sad. Here was a group of people—rich, middle-class, poor—who were connected by one thing: the inability of doctors to alleviate their symptoms. Often, their employers were unsympathetic. On my Facebook feed, amid sunny updates about vacations in Hawaii and toddlers doing funny things to cats, I would get posts like this one:

It's so frustrating that I have such good days, then I wake up and out of no where I feel like death. I'm sad, my head hurts and I feel like I could cry and I'm angry with everyone. I call it my "black hole." . . . I'm in the "black hole" now, honestly I've learned how to hide it from everyone. How truly sad is that?

Another person posted this to the group Hashimoto's 411:

I can't do this any more, I am beside myself and can't stop crying. Today, I received a disability denial letter from Social Security stating that my condition is not severe enough to qualify. . . . I don't know what to do, I feel like I am no longer living but just existing and miserable because I feel so sick. My unemployment extended benefits are going to run out and then we'll be in big trouble if we can't pay our bills, which include lots of medical bills because I don't have insurance. I just don't want to be here any more, and think my husband would be better off not having to deal with me, and with my life insurance he would be much better off financially.

The people posting questions often had multiple autoimmune diseases—each slowly developing, in sequence, like a garden coming into terrible bloom. *Is this my future?* I wondered.

But many posts also gave me hope. Online, scores of people who had had MS or rheumatoid arthritis or Hashimoto's (one of them a doctor, Terry Wahls, who eventually published a book about her findings) reported that through diet they had halted or even reversed the progression of their disease.

What I had to do, according to those who counseled these interventions, was muster the willpower to change my life. Thyroid hormone supplements were just a Band-Aid. The root cause of the autoimmune activity in my body lay elsewhere, and failing to address it meant that I might get sicker. According to many members of my Facebook group, that cause was an immune system thrown off by toxins, infections, stress, lack of sleep, and gut problems caused by an inflammatory diet—also known as "SAD," or the Standard American Diet—which had led to a proliferation of "bad" bacteria and unidentified food sensitivities. Since I got headaches when I ate, I didn't need much convincing on the food front.

At the end of June, I bowed out of a summer teaching job in Paris because I felt too sick to work. I would use the month off to focus on healing and be back in shape by the fall to resume teaching. Jim and I drove to a friend's house in Greenport on Long Island, where we often went on vacation. A historic seaport on the North Fork, Greenport is the kind of charming town with a restaurant on the dock hosting live bands and a vintage carousel running on the town green. Like me, Jim is a journalist and can work from anywhere. Being away seemed like it would offer the kind of quiet recuperative space I needed.

Jim had a busy month of deadlines, and I was trying to rest. With nothing else to distract me, I decided to embark on a diet that many people online were enthusiastic about. It was a version of the autoimmune Paleo diet, which looks a lot like the so-called Paleo regimen: no gluten, no refined sugar, little or no dairy, lots of organic meat and vegetables, but also no eggs or nightshade vegetables. The goal of the diet was to fix any underlying "gut flora dysbiosis"—an imbalance of good and bad bacteria in your gut—and begin repairing the gut by allowing the mucosal wall that lines it to heal. Along the way, I would try to figure out if I had any food sensitivities contributing to my poor health, by eliminating foods and reintroducing them one by one while observing their effects on my body.

Today, the idea that the gut plays a role in our health is familiar. But at the time, no doctor I had seen had ever mentioned the microbiome—

the community of organisms that live with us. Still, what I was reading made sense: there are both good and bad bacteria in our gut, and an imbalance of them can be a root cause of all kinds of autoimmune diseases and chronic inflammation. For example, a chronically ill person might have too much of the bacterium *Candida albicans,* which causes yeast infections and can contribute to inflammation, making you feel tired and achy. "Inflammation" is a word that gets thrown around a lot. Generally speaking, it describes what happens when immune cells detect a problem and release something known as "inflammatory mediators," which cause blood cells and immune cells to rush, say, to a wound. This process can produce pain, irritate nerves, and damage tissues. While acute inflammation is useful in helping heal wounds and fight infections, chronic inflammation is harmful to the body and has been associated with a higher risk of cancer and stroke, among other issues.

On a call with Dr. E, I asked her what she thought about the gut affecting autoimmunity. "We now know that the intestine is basically one long organ of the immune system," she said. "The gut is a tube carrying things through your body and back out. It's reasonable to think that damage to it could cause immunological problems."

By now I knew that the higher dosage of my thyroid hormone replacement hadn't gotten rid of my symptoms. The summer was lush and warm and full of possibility. But every morning I woke up feeling as if I had the flu—which I understood was a sign that my body was experiencing inappropriate inflammation. I would go outside to jump on a trampoline (supposedly it stimulates the lymphatic system, which helps eliminate toxins and waste), then come inside to dry-brush my body with a natural-bristle brush (more lymphatic benefits). For breakfast, I would pull out a container of dairy-free kefir, made from coconut—the probiotics were supposed to be good for the gut. I would mix it with cinnamon (my insulin was low, and cinnamon is said to help stabilize blood sugar) and ground flaxseed (for the omega fatty acids, which apparently reduce inflammation). Then came the almond milk, which I had to make myself. (My online advisers forbade the store-bought kind, which contained additives like carrageenan or xanthan gum.) This involved soaking the almonds overnight, pinching the skins off them one by one, grinding the nuts, pouring water through the meal—are you still with me?—and straining the liquid through an organic, unbleached cheesecloth. Next, I would add two walnuts—although I had read that they contained the wrong omega-6 to omega-3 ratios, so one had to be careful with them—and some raspberries, though I worried about the raspberries, too. They were rich in liver-protective rheosmin but also contained fructose and supposedly could ferment in the gut, encouraging the bad bacteria that led to hormone imbalances. Finally, I would sit down to eat the concoction. In this time Jim would have made coffee, read the *Times*, finished the crossword puzzle, eaten half a doughnut, and had a bowl of sugar-coated cereal. His skin seemed to glow with health.

I spent at least half of each day shopping for food, cooking, and cleaning up. I also spent many hundreds of dollars I couldn't really afford on groceries. (Nondairy kefir doesn't come cheap.) I fretted over whether it was OK to eat raw spinach, given that it may be goitrogenic (suppressive of thyroid function); hot peppers, because they're a nightshade vegetable; or eggs, because they contain lysozyme, an enzyme that—well, it's complicated.

My symptoms persisted for a couple of weeks. Then, after three weeks of the strict food regimen, the fog started to lift. If I stayed completely away from gluten—which made me feel awful, I found—I could eat without getting a headache or walk around town with Jim without needing to stop and sit down. Soon my blood pressure was close to normal. Five weeks in, I went out for a walk. Feeling unusually buoyant, I broke into a jog and found myself amid a mild endorphin rush. How I missed my old self! Please, I whispered to the sky, let this energy stay. Whatever caused it, let it stay.

When I returned to Brooklyn in August, my friend Gina emailed to invite me to dinner but wrote, "I'm afraid to cook for you!" What I had wasn't just an illness now; it was an identity, a membership in a peculiarly demanding sect. I had joined the First Assembly of the Diffusely Unwell. The Church of Fatigue, Itching, and Random Neuralgia. Temple Beth Ill. I took to asking friends if they would meet me at the one restaurant I had deemed safe, a vegan and gluten-free spot with a refrigerator full of alkalizing soup and chia-seed porridge, both unexpectedly delicious. (Or maybe it was just that I could eat them.)

Mired in the exile of my self-care, I was worried that my friends would slowly drift away. They were in their thirties, could drink, stay up late, go to parties—unlike me. I watched the lives of others with a sense of wistfulness. I missed the burn of Scotch in my throat, the loose joy of a dinner party where everyone got a little high on talk. I wanted to be sloppy and fun again. "How are you doing?" Gina asked one morning. "I don't know if I can take this anymore," I told her. "I just want to get better. I want to go for a day without *thinking* about my body."

But the restrictive program I had myself on seemed my best chance at recovery. In New York, I started seeing a nutritionist who performed a kind of energy-based muscle testing. She put me on supplements that helped me feel better. (Placebo effect? I didn't care.) Another practitioner gave me a silver solution to boost my immune system and soothe my sore throat. I knew that I was a mark for any faddist who came along, but I tried to chart my symptoms, to treat myself like a lab subject.

In the late weeks of that summer of 2012, as the fall semester approached, I prepared for my classes with a new sense of focus. I felt sorry for the previous me, who had labored self-consciously to teach, feeling stupid, just because her thyroid was not working.

When I went back to my doctor in September to have my thyroid levels retested, my thyroid hormones were still out of whack, but my destructive autoantibodies were gone. I was on my way back to wellness, I thought.

. . .

IF I'D HAD A DIFFERENT kind of disease, my story would end here. But the nature of many immune-modulated or inflammatory disorders is to attack in cycles, to flare. One morning not long after that doctor visit, I couldn't get out of bed. For two weeks, I woke up with aches and a fever. It was a struggle to do anything—to teach my class, to clean the house. I had nosebleeds and large bruises. My blood pressure dropped again, and one day when I got out of bed I fainted, gashing my arm on a glass on the night table. When I came to, I was on the ground, shards of glass around me, a maroon swoop of murky blood dripping across my forearm.

What is happening to me? I wondered. I came across Jim googling "symptoms of leukemia" at our kitchen table. He shrugged when I asked him what he was doing. "You don't seem well," he said quietly.

I made my way to my doctor's busy office, crossing long avenues in the rain from the 4 train to the hospital by the East River, and sat in the waiting room, my pants still damp, with people who looked very sick. When I raised concerns about how I was doing, Dr. E told me gently, "You may need to adjust to the fact that you're not the same as you once were. You may always feel like you're eighty percent." She intended, I know, to help me adjust to a new reality, but the effect was the opposite. The prospect was unbearable. I deflated like a punctured pool float. As a nurse drew my blood, I stared at the test tubes, wishing that the purplish red liquid filling them could yield a definitive explanation for my remaining symptoms.

A few days later, Dr. E called while I was out for a walk. "Your labs look normal, except for the thyroid hormones." She explained that the blood work showed an unusual pattern of hormones, some of which looked mildly low, others of which indicated that I could be overmedicated. "Perhaps you should try lowering your dose. You might be hyperthyroid now."

I told her it felt as if I needed to raise the dose—my limbs were like heavy weights.

"OK, then, raise the dose and see how you do," she said agreeably.

I was both grateful—I'd found a doctor who took my input seriously—and unnerved. Even this expert physician did not know what was happening in my body. Like many patients, I hungered for cast-iron certainty even though I realized that I was living in a morass of uncertainty—why was I always iron and vitamin D deficient? Why was it so hard to treat my disease? I found myself wishing I could have blood tests every few months, to chart my antibodies and vitamin levels.

I had other causes for concern: I was in near constant pain, and my right thumb and left foot were almost entirely numb. On some days, I couldn't open jars or sign my name on checks. I saw a neurologist about the electric shocks, and she told me that she thought my body might now be attacking the small fibers of my nervous system. *You're not imagining it,* she said kindly. *We just might not be able to do anything to help you.* Her kindness—and her acknowledgment that I was suffering from *something*—buoyed me. On the long subway trip from the hospital to my apartment in Brooklyn I felt momentarily hopeful.

In the way of things, I woke the next day in pain and found myself mourning my old robust state of health. I looked at the photograph by my desk of me as a teenager and remembered playing in the sun on vacation. I remembered getting up early during those long months with the feeling that, like the boy in Robert Lowell's poem "Waking Early Sunday Morning," I sat "like a dragon on / time's hoard." I remembered going downstairs before anyone had woken to sit with my book and a bowl of cereal. Later, the dog and I would go out for a walk up the dirt road by our cabin, under the tall New England sugar maples. I'd throw the tennis ball for him, feeling the wet-cool dirt and gravel under my bare feet. I remember being so lost in the sun and the dog's joy and my pleasure in these hours of freedom that I had no sense that I lived in a body, except as a thing that could feel the sun and the wind and the dog's cold nose.

THREE

DISEASE CONCEPTS

That fall, as the leaves thinned on the trees, I found myself obsessively wondering, What does it mean to have a disease doctors can't diagnose? Why had it taken me so long to get answers in our hyperdiagnostic age, in which you can get a diagnosis for everything from shyness to sphenopalatine ganglioneuralgia (also known as "ice-cream headache")?

I settled into an uneasy equilibrium. Teaching still required an immense effort, but I could do it if I was obsessive about taking care of myself. My social life was nearly nonexistent. Most nights I stayed in with Jim and watched a TV show or a movie. The fuzzy memories I have of this time are of sitting on the couch, a chenille blanket covering our legs, as a film studio logo streamed past and I felt the flicker of promise that I'd be taken out of myself for an hour or two. Films were easier for me to watch than TV, because I found that I was increasingly unable to remember what had happened on the previous episode of a show, even when we had watched it mere days ago. "Wait, who is that again? And what happened to him?" I would ask. Jim would mumble a semi-answer, intent on the unfolding story.

When I had energy at the end of the day, which was rare, I read or worked, slowly, on class prep and my own writing. I was finding it hard to write, because my brain was so fuzzy, but I needed to make money, to pay the rent, to see doctors. Taking time off was not an option if I could still force myself on. And I loved working. Writing was how I made sense of the world; it kept me tethered to a key part of myself. To find that I was sick in a way that made any immersion in my work impossible—this was a blow for me, too, one that I couldn't accept yet. And so I sat at my desk every day, even though I often nodded off in my chair, waking myself up when my head hit the computer screen.

Occasionally Jim and I went to a party, and I had a half glass of wine, which made me feel as if I were struggling to lift my eyelids. Going to dinners with friends became so taxing, despite my hunger for company and conversation, that I rarely left my house. I didn't know how to explain to others what was going on. I appeared fine, after all. ("You *look* great," people kept saying, almost in disbelief.)

I turned up the dial on my homegrown research, spending hours online in patient groups reading about other people suffering from fatigue. (Such an empty word: it sounded like I meant I was tired, whereas I kept imagining my body's mitochondria were sick, like those of little Charles Wallace in Madeleine L'Engle's *A Wind in the Door*.) By now, I could barely summon up the energy to walk more than a few blocks. I looked for other patients who had experienced my electric shocks, but I couldn't find any in the online autoimmune patient groups, though many had variants of classic neuropathies. Soon I was buried in subreddit threads about ATP processes and the hypothalamic-pituitary-adrenal axis. The HPA axis, as I learned, is a term for the interconnected systems ("an intricate, yet robust, neuroendocrine mechanism," as one article put it) by which the body responds to and overcomes stressors, mediating the effects of everything from infections to trauma by regulating immune cells, metabolism, hormones, and the autonomic nervous system. Disorders of it could lead to all kinds of problems. I wasn't a doctor, but the more I learned about the HPA axis and the autonomic nervous system, which itself controls involuntary processes such as blood pressure, temperature regulation, and digestion, the more I suspected the possibility of a connection among my diverse symptoms.

Along the way I ordered books about adrenal fatigue, a diagnosis that is not recognized by Western medicine but that many chronically ill patients consider to be a key factor in unexplained exhaustion. The notion is that the wear and tear of modern life—or the ravages of infections—have taxed the sufferer's adrenal gland, which releases cortisol, a stress hormone, leading to disruptions in the circadian rhythm and then to insomnia and fatigue. I consulted a practitioner who tested for it, using a saliva test, and he expressed surprise at the results: my cortisol levels were close to normal. But maybe a little adrenal support (in the form of herbs) would help. I began taking licorice pills in the morning and trying to be in bed by ten p.m., in hopes of restoring my energy naturally.

In the meantime, our apartment had become my world, and I turned a consequently oversized attention to it, fussing with pillows, rearranging a bookshelf if I felt up to it, spending hours in bed browsing design sites. On other days I spent hours in bed looking at clothes. At the time this made me feel like a fraud. If I could window-shop on the internet, surely I could summon up the willpower to be writing, to be reading. Instead, I'd become someone without an inner life.

These hours of aspirational longing, I now more forgivingly think, were a response to the illness. I was trying to manifest the person I wanted to be: a person who could enjoy her life, her home, a person who wasn't about to die or disappear. The part of me that spent hours looking at home design sites and clothing on sale was the part of me that wanted to live and didn't know how else to express it. The worse I felt, the less I could do what I wanted (work, *think*), the more I searched for beauty and for pleasure.

What I didn't fully understand then was how sick I still was, thanks in part to undiagnosed infections that were contributing to a host of immunological anomalies in my body, as well as dysautonomia, or dysfunction in my autonomic nervous system. At the time, I knew only that I was a somewhat anxious young woman with largely invisible and hard-to-measure symptoms that came and went and affected different parts of my body.

And that, as it turned out, meant I was in real trouble, given the realities of the current U.S. medical system.

DISEASE HAS ALWAYS BEEN a part of human life, but how humans understand it changes. For centuries, medical practices across cultures viewed illness as a disruption of balance. Unlike modern Western medicine, these systems drew a connection between the individual constitution and the patient's treatment. "It is more important to know what sort of person has a disease than to know what sort of disease a person has," the ancient Greek physician Hippocrates is credited with having said. It was Hippocrates who advanced the theory that the body and our emotions were influenced by the four humors (blood, yellow bile, black bile, and phlegm), a theory that persisted through the Renaissance. (Shakespeare often invoked the humors in his plays.) In the East, Chinese medicine sought to harmonize the body and return its energies to a balanced state. Presented with six patients who have abdominal pain, Ted Kaptchuk, a professor of medicine at Harvard Medical School, points out in *The Web That Has No Weaver: Understanding Chinese Medicine*, "the Chinese doctor . . . distinguishes six patterns of disharmony where Western medicine perceives only one disease."

Today, Western medical science typically conceives of a disease as falling into one of three categories. The first consists of diseases with a single identifiable cause, like smallpox or strep throat—what scientists call a "specific disease entity." The second consists of diseases that are (as we might say colloquially) "all in your head"—the convictions of illness known as "conversion disorder," or plain old hypochondria, embodied by Woody Allen's character in *Hannah and Her Sisters*, who is convinced first that he has a malignant melanoma, then that he has a brain tumor. ("Do you hear a buzzing? Is there a buzzing?" he anxiously asks his secretary.) The third category encompasses diseases or conditions that are accepted as biologically real but are believed to be caused or exacerbated by stress and the mind, such as panic attacks or ulcers. (Western medicine generally treats mental illness as a fourth category altogether.)

For years, medicine has found it easiest to conceive of the first and second categories: assigning some conditions to the category of measurable "real" disease while labeling others psychosomatic diseases best treated by a psychiatrist. But something like autoimmune disease or long COVID falls into the third category of illness; it combines biology and biography in ways that are difficult for most of us (whether scientists or laypeople) to conceptualize. As the medical historian Charles Rosenberg asserts, "There is no simple, one-dimensional way to understand those entities we call autoimmune diseases." Autoimmune diseases have biological markers, but they come and go, and patients' flares can be exacerbated by stress. Such diseases require us to think about illness in a more complex way than we usually do, a more complex way than twentieth-century medicine did, since it was, at heart, based on the idea that all bodies respond roughly the same way to infection. That perspective is turning out to be oversimplified.

The old framework dates to the nineteenth-century embrace of germ theory: the idea that infectious diseases are caused by a single observable pathogen, which produces distinct and predictable symptoms. Germ theory had a dramatic clarity to it. It pushed Western medicine away from an earlier holistic emphasis on the role an individual's constitution played in illness and toward the measuring of the effects produced by a specific germ. In 1890, the German bacteriologist Robert

Koch laid out a strict set of rules, known as "Koch's postulates," about what constituted an infectious disease, relying on the idea that bacteria would affect everyone pretty much the same way. The result was a tidy vision of disease in which "each species of germ is supposed to incite one type of disease and elicit perfectly matched antibodies," as Anderson and Mackay write in *Intolerant Bodies*. Focus shifted from the soil to the seed, as it were.

Giving doctors tools to cure formerly hard-to-treat illnesses, germ theory ushered in a golden era of professionalized medicine—and bacteriology. "Having heard of microbes much as Saint Thomas Aquinas heard of angels," George Bernard Shaw wrote in the preface to his 1906 play *The Doctor's Dilemma*, a generation of doctors "suddenly concluded that the whole art of healing could be summed up in the formula: find the microbe and kill it." Around the same time, advances in lab testing and new technologies like the X-ray helped legitimate "this newly specific way of thinking about disease," as Rosenberg puts it, transforming medicine from a healing-oriented moral practice into a diagnosis-oriented science focused on discernible, and replicable, test results. By 1932, the historian Henry E. Sigerist had noted that medicine's systemizing impulses were "no longer concerned with man but with disease," as Anderson and Mackay point out.

This pivot was, in many ways, a good thing: it increased survival rates from infectious diseases and gave us longer lives on average. But it had one particularly negative consequence: doctors began to question whether illnesses they could not readily measure on tests were real. They doubted the testimony of those with amorphous illnesses such as autoimmunity, ME/CFS, or fibromyalgia, for which there is not always an easy test, an identifiable cause, or an effective treatment. Today, a doctor presented with a hard-to-identify disease will often shrug the patient off, and so patients who report lingering symptoms after an infection, for example, have long been ignored or dismissed when initial tests failed to turn up anything. As Susan Block, a Harvard professor of psychiatry and medicine, and a pioneer of palliative care, told me, "The tendency in many parts of medicine is, if we can't measure it, it doesn't exist, or the patient is cuckoo."

In recent years, though, medical pioneers have pushed past the "if we can't measure it, it doesn't exist" view, bringing the individual constitution (the soil) back into consideration and articulating a more sophisticated idea: that the immune system's response to a pathogen could be what does much of the damage to our bodies. This new paradigm holds that disease is a multipronged phenomenon—an interaction among pathogens, the immune system, and the "environment," a term that can refer to a person's microbiome or exposure to such things as toxic chemicals and trauma. (Both have been shown to affect the immune system.)

At the vanguard of an emerging personalized medicine, this new view of illness recognizes that individual immune responses to infections vary dramatically and are influenced by social and genetic determinants of health. In fact, it now appears that a host of different infections may trigger long-term illness in certain patients. A 2018 study conducted by researchers at the Cincinnati Children's Hospital showed that Epstein-Barr virus, which can develop into mononucleosis, increases the risk of lupus in a genetically susceptible group of people. Researchers at Stanford and Columbia are exploring immune pathways by which certain infections (for example, strep throat) can trigger PANS (pediatric acute-onset neuropsychiatric syndrome) in some children. And now, of course, there's COVID.

COVID-19 is a test case for this new model of thinking about infection as a trigger of immune dysfunction. One of the disease's great mysteries is why some thirty-year-olds die from it and others don't even notice they have it, while still others have a mild acute case but end up suffering from long COVID for months afterward, unable to walk up a flight of stairs without getting winded and dizzy. This pandemic has vividly dramatized the variability—and lingering complexity—of the human host's response to a pathogen.

"This is something that has been going on forever," Craig Spencer, the director of global health in emergency medicine at Columbia University, says about the variability of human response to infection. "I wouldn't be surprised if people are walking about with long Epstein-Barr virus, or long influenza. We all know someone who is low energy, who's told to work harder. We have all heard about chronic Lyme sufferers, and those with ME/CFS. But they get written off." Spencer understands something about how infections can do long-term damage, because he contracted Ebola while working in Guinea, fell ill upon his return to New York City, and then struggled with the virus's ongoing effects. (Studies have suggested that the Ebola virus may linger in the body for years.)

The difference between long COVID and other infection-associated illnesses is that it is happening "on such a huge scale—unlike anything we've seen before. It is harder for the medical community to write off," Spencer told me. Indeed, many researchers I spoke with for this book hope that the race to understand long COVID will advance our understanding of other chronic conditions that follow infection, transforming medicine in the process.

To UNDERSTAND THE CONCEPTUAL CHALLENGE facing medicine as it grapples with long COVID and other infection-associated diseases, it may be helpful to look at the evolution of our understanding of a very different condition: ulcers. Ulcers, famously, were once thought of as a purely psychological phenomenon—caused by stress. The 1943 manual *Understand Your Ulcer* informs patients that ulcers are "a disease of tense, nervous people who lead a strenuous and worrisome life." As recently as 1983, many physicians thought of ulcers as "a darkly self-inflicted wound" or a result of the "tense tempo of modern life," as Terence Monmaney reported in *The New Yorker*.

Then, in 1979, an Australian pathologist at the Royal Perth Hospital found something that surprised him: bacteria in the biopsies of stomach tissue taken from patients with digestive complaints. At the time, an indisputable tenet of medicine held that the stomach was a sterile environment—no bacteria lived inside it. Intrigued by the pathologist's unusual finding, a microbiologist named Barry Marshall (also at Perth) began studying biopsies. And in the tissue from biopsies of patients with peptic ulcers and stomach inflammation, he found bacteria—corkscrew-shaped microbes one hundredth the size of a grain of sand. In 1983, Marshall presented his surprising findings to a meeting of infectious disease specialists, only to be met with ridicule. Critics countered that obviously the bacteria Marshall had seen were from contaminated surfaces or had opportunistically colonized the stomach after an ulcer had weakened its lining. Their fierce response was a classic example of what is known as the "Semmelweis reflex"—the reflexive rejection of new paradigms in medicine.

To prove he was right, Marshall decided to take a dramatic step: he infected himself by drinking a vial containing millions of the bacteria he had found in sick patients' stomachs. A week or so later, he began vomiting. His breath smelled sour. He grew irritable and tired, and he was often hungry. A follow-up endoscopy found that his formerly healthy pink stomach tissue was now "punky" (as Monmaney puts it) and that bacteria appeared to "swarm" around "inflamed stomach cells." A few days later, Marshall began to feel better. A third endoscopy showed that his tissue looked fine. His immune system had fended off the bacteria. But he had evidence that they had, for a time, made him sick.

Marshall named the bacterium *Helicobacter pylori*. Researchers began replicating his findings. A decade later, in 1993, *The Wall Street Journal* trumpeted, "Studies Confirm Most Ulcers Are Caused by a Bacterium, Curable by Antibiotics." Furthermore, in some people the bacterial infection went on to cause stomach cancer—showing that an infection could be a trigger for cancer.

The news ushered in a revolution in the conception and treatment of ulcers. By 1997, as Michael Specter reported in *The New Yorker*, a prominent gastroenterologist would declare, "The only good *Helicobacter pylori* is a dead *Helicobacter pylori*."

Ulcers, then, went from being seen as a disease that was caused by stress to a disease that was caused by a bacterium. But the story didn't end there. It now seems that while *H. pylori* does trigger ulcers, they can be compounded by stress, for reasons that are not well understood. More important, *H. pylori* doesn't trigger ulcers in everyone. In fact, when researchers started testing for *H. pylori*, they found that it infects around two thirds of the world's population, many of whom did not have ulcers. But the coverage of Marshall's triumphal discovery left this out of the account and never asked one obvious question: If the infection is so common, why isn't it giving *everyone* who has it ulcers? Why do some people get ulcers and not others? The seed had been shown to be invasive, but some soil, like Marshall's, seemed resilient enough to fend it off. Instead of publicly considering these questions, medicine swung from one kind of appealingly conventional explanation (it's psychological) to another (a bacterium causes it).

Today, medicine has come to understand ulcers in a third way, as a disease that seems to be triggered by a complex interplay between bacterium and host. In fact, there is some truth to the notion that ulcers are associated with anxiety: stress, or an unknown variable correlated with it, can make *H. pylori* infections worse, as if it transforms the bacterium in certain instances from a neutral force to a pathological one. On its own, *H. pylori* is not malevolent: it often lives with us in what's called a "commensal" relationship, in which two species coexist without harm, or even benefit from their coexistence. One study found that *H. pylori* may even play a positive role in human health: adults without it in their stomachs are more likely to have suffered from asthma as children. But under certain conditions, the host's physiology changes, and the benign relationship evolves into a pathological one.

THE STORY OF ULCERS SHOWS that the premodern notion of a disease as an imbalance in an individual's homeostatic system still has something to offer us, though such personalized approaches were largely rejected when Western medicine embraced germ theory. Today, as a new paradigm for disease is emerging—pushed into full view by the coronavirus pandemic—we must amend the simple "germ causes disease, body overcomes disease" model. In some people, a germ can have little or moderate effect. In others, it can trigger a cascade of ongoing effects in the body that persist after the initial acute infection; perhaps, too, more infections linger in the body than we had previously realized. Complicating germ theory's paradigm of a specific disease entity, or the infection that tidily resolves, researchers are showing that much of health depends on the interplay between soil and seed, host and infection, with the immune system and one's microbiome as confounding factors. And so autoimmune disease and immune-mediated diseases necessitate a more holistic and personalized understanding of disease and immunity than conventional germ theory offered. As Charles Rosenberg notes, they require "an older way of thinking about the fundamental nature of disease, a way of thinking that was commonplace in 1800 but marginal by 2000."

Ironically, other aspects of modernity, from antibiotics to processed diets to an explosive growth of chemicals in the environment, may have contributed to a vast increase in these diseases precisely when medicine was evolving to embrace one-size-fits-all diagnoses. Today, to treat the growing numbers of patients living with these amorphous, system-roaming illnesses, medicine may need to return to a model of disease at the core of ancient medicine, one that sees sickness as a disruption of a particular body's natural balance.

One useful model for how variability works is the idea of the "allostatic load," a term coined in 1993 by Bruce McEwen, a neuroendocrinologist at Rockefeller University, and Eliot Stellar, a psychologist at the University of Pennsylvania, to denote the weight of the wear and tear on a body as it tries to retain equilibrium in a taxing and stressful world. The lower an individual's allostatic load, the easier it is for that person's body to stay healthy. The higher it is—because the person lives in a polluted area, has an infection, suffers food insecurity, or lives with a chronic stressor such as systemic racism—the likelier you are to get sick with various diseases. But in the early years of a disease process, the system's metabolic strain may not appear in lab work as abnormal results. It takes a discerning doctor to interpret early variations that are signs of disease and to point out the trajectory the patient's body is on.

Thinking about disease as a complex individualized consequence of genes and infections and stress and our immune systems means living with uncertainty instead of diagnostic clarity. The twentieth century was, as Sontag put it, "an era in which medicine's central premise is that all diseases can be cured." The twenty-first century will be an era in which medicine embraces the complexity of disease triggers. Our illness narratives accordingly must evolve from accounts of dramatic onset and ultimate cure (or tragic death) to subtler accounts of change. In this model, many of us may live in a gray area between health and disease for years, amorphously fluctuating between feeling well and being symptomatic.

In the meantime, modern medicine's stigmatization of patients who lack clear-cut test results continues to be a chief shortcoming of the American health care system, which, in its understandable embrace of authoritative answers, struggles to acknowledge what it does not know.

In *Arrowsmith*, his novel about early-twentieth-century medicine's ardor for the laboratory, the novelist Sinclair Lewis identified the ways germ theory had led to an outsized faith in measurement. The protagonist's mentor, a German-accented bacteriologist named Max Gottlieb, stands beside his test tubes and his microscope and declares that the authentic scientist is a revolutionary *precisely* "because he alone knows how liddle he knows." I read the book one day in bed and found myself wondering how many people today are suffering unrecognized and largely alone because modern medicine is bad at acknowledging "how liddle" it knows. I felt a prickle at the special horror of being not only ill but also marginalized—your testimony dismissed because your lab work fails to match a preexisting pattern.

FOUR

IMPERSONATION

One of the hardest things about being ill with a poorly understood disease is that most people find what you're going through incomprehensible—if they even believe you *are* going through it. In your loneliness, your preoccupation with an enduring new reality, you want to be understood in a way that you can't be. "Pain is always new to the sufferer, but loses its originality for those around him," Alphonse Daudet observes in *In the Land of Pain*. "Everyone will get used to it except me."

Worrying that your symptoms are psychosomatic—or even imagined— is part of life for many people with poorly understood illnesses. Although the experience of illness is not just in the head, it is also not just in the body. The person enduring such an illness faces a difficult balancing act. On the one hand, she must advocate for herself, even when doctors are indifferent or ignorant, and not be deterred when she knows something is wrong. On the other, she also must be willing to ask whether an obsessive attention to symptoms is going to lead to better health. The patient has to hold in mind two contradictory modes, in other words: insistence on the reality of the disease and resistance to her own catastrophic fears. I found it hard, in the fall and winter of 2012, to strike that balance. I was increasingly worried.

After all, a terrible anxiety attends chronic illness. Over time, it becomes difficult to untangle the suffering from symptoms like pain from the suffering inflicted by the anxiety over the possibility of more pain, and worse outcomes, in the future. This does not mean that the illness is in the mind; rather, the mind—that machine for making meaning—makes endless meanings of its new state, which may themselves influence the experience.

It was in this recursive hall of mirrors, trying to adjust to my body's ailments, that I lived.

There is a loneliness to illness, a child's desire to be pitied and seen. But it is precisely this recognition that is elusive. How can you explain and identify your condition if no one has any grasp of what it is you suffer from and the symptoms wax and wane? How do you describe a disease that's not always there?

The hardest thing to convey to doctors or friends was the debilitating fatigue, which many other patients I knew experienced as well. Complaining of fatigue sounds like moral weakness; in New York City, tired is normal. But the fatigue of physical dysfunction, I came to recognize, is as different from normal sleep deprivation as COVID-19 is from the common cold. It was not caused by needing sleep, I thought, but by my body's cellular conviction that it needed to conserve energy in order to fix whatever was wrong. The feeling erased my will, the sense of identity that drives most of us. The worst part of my fatigue was the loss of an intact sense of self.

It wasn't just that I suffered brain fog; it wasn't just the loss of self that sociologists talk about in connection with chronic illness, in which everything you know about yourself disappears and you have to build a different life. Rather, as I got sicker that winter, I no longer had the sense that I was a distinct person. On most days, I felt like a mechanism that moved arduously through the world simply trying to complete its tasks. Sitting upright at my father's birthday dinner at a quiet restaurant required a huge act of will. Normally, absorption in a task—an immersive flow—can lead you to forget that you feel pain, but my fatigue made such a state impossible. I might, at the nadir of my illness, have been able to write any one of these sentences, but I would not have been able to make paragraphs of them.

To be sick in this way is to have the unpleasant feeling that you are impersonating yourself. When you're sick, the act of living is more act than living. Healthy people have the luxury of forgetting that their existence depends on a cascade of precise cellular interactions. Not you. "Farewell me, cherished me, now so hazy, so indistinct," Daudet writes—a line I now often thought of.

My mental sensation of no longer being a person had a correlating physical symptom: my eyes no longer seemed like lenses onto the world. They seemed, rather, to be distinct parts of my body, as perceptible as fingers—oddly distant, protuberant, like old-fashioned spectacles. My face was a mask I was conscious of at all times. It made me feel categorically fraudulent. I could feel the fat in my cheeks and the weight of my bones as I spoke. I experienced a mounting anxiety: everything was wrong, and that wrongness was inside me, but I wasn't sure anymore who that "me" was, or how to express what was happening.

As Virginia Woolf testified in *On Being Ill*, "English, which can express the thoughts of Hamlet and the tragedy of Lear, has no words for the shiver and the headache. . . . The merest schoolgirl, when she falls in love, has Shakespeare or Keats to speak her mind for her; but let a sufferer try to describe a pain in his head to a doctor and language at once runs dry."

For me the hardest part was not being comprehended, or not believed. "Physical pain does not simply resist language but actively destroys it," writes Elaine Scarry in *The Body in Pain*. "To have pain is to have *certainty*; to hear about pain is to have *doubt*." The same was true of all my symptoms, none of which could be seen.

In those months I was lonely in a way I never had been before. I could taste the solitude of the human body like brine in my mouth, a taste that never left me.

I WAS THIRTY-SIX WHEN I realized that not everyone in their twenties and thirties was in pain all the time. I had been in pain of one sort or another since college, much of it muscular or joint pain, some of it gynecological. In 2011, I started having serious hip pain and was diagnosed with a torn labrum and arthritis, for which I had surgery that I was slow to recover from. By 2012, when I came to understand I was sick, pain was only one of my symptoms, and not even the worst. But its constancy was wearing. It moved around my body, changing from day to day, worse one day in my hips, the next my neck or my right thumb. My muscles were always tight; shooting pains ran from my shoulder to my neck, or down my legs.

Some days, the pain tipped from manageable to consuming, as if my brain had been caught in an unexpected electrical storm. When it did, it was as if a high-pitched noise no one else could hear was in the room. It distracted me and made me irritable. I was both present with others and off in my head, attending to the pain, trying to gauge its neural contours. One day, pulling down a box of sweaters from a high shelf, I felt pain radiate through my neck and back, which froze up. X-rays found that I had cervical spine scoliosis, compression of a cervical disc (likely the cause of my acute pain), and extensive arthritis in my neck; the doctor, who knew about my hip, mused that I was having a lot of issues with my connective tissue. I started physical therapy, where I had to rank my pain level on a scale of 1 to 10 week after week, an exercise I found impossible: How to describe intermittent severe pain on the same scale as constant middle-range pain, which I found more debilitating? Attempting to reduce pain that was context dependent to a number just made it clear that there was no way to make this invisible symptom legible to others. And the poet in me found all the metaphors for pain to be limited. "Burning," "tingling," "stabbing"—these words did little to describe pain's reality, which ebbed and flowed according to its own logic. Pain was an empire of its own, well defended against language's forays against it.

At the urging of first one friend, then another, I read everything I could by John Sarno, a New York physician who had written several best-selling books about his conviction that a great deal of back, neck, shoulder, and carpal tunnel pain is caused by repressed negative emotions—such as stress, anger, and anxiety—in people inclined to bottle things up. He argued that these repressed emotions can cause muscle pain by reducing blood flow to the area in question, leading to a syndrome he termed "tension myositis syndrome" (TMS). Sarno, who died in 2017, believed that if such patients acknowledge and exorcise their negative emotions, their pain will disappear, because it is the body's way of distracting the mind from a trauma or source of anguish. Open to anything, I did what he advised, wondering if in fact I suffered from repressed anger. Could it be that something like my ongoing grief at my mother's death was the real problem?

But none of Sarno's exercises worked for me—though I went so far as to see a therapist trained in his methods. I grew frustrated that so many people wanted to assume that my pain was emotional in origin without knowing anything about my medical history. The idea that emotional tension could lead to pain struck me as logical based on my limited understanding of biology, but it also seemed to me that some people embraced Sarno's framework as yet another way of finding certainty where uncertainty lived. Usually, it became clear that Sarno's approach had been a magic solution for them. (It had worked for them; therefore it must work for *you*—a mindset one encounters a lot.) I suspected that something more complicated was going on, and that I was not yet done with uncertainty.

All I knew was that day after day the pain moved around. I did my best to ignore it.

MY FATHER, WHO WAS JUST emerging from a period of acute mourning for my mother, lived in a small town in Connecticut, about ninety minutes from Brooklyn, where my parents had moved in 2003 so that my mother could become the head of a local private school. My father ran the languages department there. Jim and I saw him periodically for dinner, sometimes with my brothers, Liam and Eamon, who also lived in Brooklyn. I told him that I wasn't feeling well, but in the absence of an identifiable illness, what was he supposed to say or do? "I'm sorry you're feeling so bad," he once said to me on the phone, in his indirect Irish American way, apropos of nothing. Today, I hear the empathy and helplessness he must have felt, but at the time the concern felt remote.

I was beginning to confront the fact that the Hashimoto's diagnosis, though crucial, did not explain my ongoing poor health. As my doctor had noted enthusiastically at a recent visit, the lab work showed my autoantibodies were still almost nonexistent. The thyroid medication had normalized my hormone levels. I should be feeling well. Neither she nor any other doctor was able to give a name to my ongoing illlness; it was invisible, vague. My brothers were sympathetic but busy with their own lives, still wrestling with the aftermath of our mother's death. It was shocking to me how much I missed her, how much worse it was to be sick without her comfort and counsel. At times I thought I would slowly slip away unseen and no one would notice because the shell of my body was still there.

One night I went to a work event in the West Village, at which people I hadn't seen for months were dressed in party clothes—sheen of silk, bare shoulders, men in leather shoes—smoking on the balcony. "How are you feeling, Meghan?" a tall poet asked, putting his hand on my shoulder in genuine concern, a cigarette dangling between his lips. "Meghan!" cried two others I hadn't seen in a year, leaning languorously against the balcony wall in a way that made me nervous. What was there to say? It was New York City; everybody was striving to feel more, be more. I had the sensation that I needed to find a better story to tell about my condition, because of course I had no story at all. In her poignant memoir *A Body, Undone*, about a bike accident that left her largely paralyzed, the scholar Christina Crosby writes, "Whenever you offer an account of yourself to others, you labor to present yourself as coherent and worthy of recognition and attention, as I am doing right now."

This labor was precisely what I was failing to perform; in my fatigue and pain I couldn't find the words to make myself legible to others. (And I still have not found them. This text is full of silences and vagueness and lacunae: when I write "brain fog," I imagine that your mind slides over the idea, unless you, too, have suffered from it.) In the absence of that recognition, I began to see myself as not only incoherent but also unworthy, ashamed that I craved comfort from others.

I chatted on the balcony, sorrow growing in me, then went inside and got my coat to go home.

IN THIS PERIOD, I did find comfort in books. In bits and pieces, I was reading poetry I loved, and trying to write poems, too. I managed to write a few short essays I was proud of. But it was often almost impossible to read. Usually, I fell asleep trying, the light from my bedside lamp warm on my left cheek, the dark purple walls of our tiny Brooklyn bedroom cocooning me as buses roared past, taking people to and from their jobs.

In those late fall months, I lived as if in a locked room. I could only look out the windows, catching fragmentary glimpses of life as I'd once enjoyed it, growing even more determined to find answers.

Outside, my friends were meeting in the park, eating picnic lunches in sweaters as their children poked one another with sticks, or hailing taxis in a sudden downpour, giving the stranger at a party a second, hungry look.

Inside, it was dark and stuffy, and I labored to survive an illness no one could see. In this way the undiagnosed suffer, doubly alone.

At times I thought the only way to escape was to become mad, like the narrator of Charlotte Perkins Gilman's "The Yellow Wall-paper," who goes slowly insane when her husband, a physician, treats her case of "a slight hysterical tendency" (brought on by the birth of her son) by keeping her locked in a room on the top floor of a house they have leased.

I would have to make a window in my experience through which I could climb out, whatever that meant.

Why does a diagnosis matter so much to you? a friend asked me at one point.

I know many people who are suspicious of diagnoses—they think of them as labels that reduce or stigmatize. I knew, already, that a diagnosis was not going to answer all my questions. But I craved a diagnosis because it is a form of understanding.

Knowledge brings the hope of treatment or cure. And even if there is no cure, a diagnosis is a form of knowing (the word "diagnosis" derives from the Greek *gignōskein*, "to know") that allows others to recognize our experience and enables us to tell its story. I felt acutely the absence of a story I could tell others. Without a story, who—or what—would help me get better?

ALICE JAMES, William and Henry's sister, was sick from adolescence on with a disease no one could exactly name or treat (though she was diagnosed with hysteria). Near the end of her life, when she was finally given a breast cancer diagnosis, she rejoiced in her diary, "To him who waits, all things come! . . . Ever since I have been ill, I have longed and longed for some palpable disease, no matter how conventionally dreadful a label it might have." Anyone who has suffered from an unnamed illness can understand the perversity of the logic. At last, James writes, she was released from "the monstrous mass of subjective sensations," which "that 'medical man' had no higher inspiration than to assure me I was personally responsible for, washing his hands of me with graceful complacency." She died of breast cancer within a year of the diagnosis. So challenging was living with an unidentified illness that she welcomed the terrible news with what sounds like excitement.

When I read this in her diary, on a brisk October night, I set the book down. The night's shadows had lengthened, the streetlamps with their sodium glow brightened the darkness beyond. I couldn't pinpoint what was disturbing me, except that it had to do with the waste of this life and this mind.

Sitting on my couch, I felt Alice James's shadow inside me. I knew what it felt like to have your illness go unnamed. I could imagine what it was like to give up, to feel your mind go as wobbly as your body, reconciling yourself to the idea that death would really be a relief—a respite from lonely suffering. I could sense, inside my body, the muddled pains of hers.

It was also all too easy for me to imagine how the nineteenth-century conception of hysteria led her to assume that her symptoms were her own personal failings. I felt a wasteland of sorrow. Too much of my own life had been spent wondering if what was wrong with me was a deficiency of character. I also felt fear: Would my doctors assume, as her doctors had of Alice, that some mental strife was the source of my disease—a dis-ease, in other words?

This was why I wanted others to see what was happening to me, to *know* that I was locked away in the room alone. If they knew, perhaps someone could find a way to get me out. Instead, I feared, I would be relegated to a world of the imaginary ill, exiled to an invisible kingdom from which I would never be allowed passage.

My testimony wasn't doing the job. ("You *look* great.")

Yet I felt deeply that *something was wrong.* I can't put this into clinical language. All I can say is that it was a bone-deep, a cell-deep conviction: that whatever was wrong *was not* in my head. The symptoms—roving neurological pain, headaches, flu-like aches, sensitivity to food—were too specific. And my lab work had so many small clues. Low vitamin D. Anemia. The many viruses.

Where was the scientist, the doctor, who felt acutely "how liddle he knows" and would come to help me, to help all of us in this condition?

I knew such doctors were out there, and at night I prayed for them to succeed.

Please, I thought, *know that we are here and we need your help.*

FIVE

THE DOCTOR-PATIENT
RELATIONSHIP

In the fall and winter of 2012, debt piled up as I continued to seek out top-tier physicians, many of whom did not accept insurance. As several told me, the costly bureaucratic requirements imposed by insurance companies got in the way of spending time with their patients. I saw a rheumatologist who dictated his notes in front of me ("Patient in midthirties with a pleasing affect . . .") and told me I had an antigen called HLA-B27, associated with ankylosing spondylitis (an autoimmune disease), and recommended follow-up MRIs, which led nowhere. Another doctor I saw, I could tell, wasn't sure what to think when he heard me say that fatigue and brain fog were my worst symptoms. *Is this all in her head?* I imagined him wondering. One suggested I see a therapist. The trouble was not that he was suggesting I seek mental health care—I had seen excellent therapists. Counseling plays a crucial supportive role in the management of chronic illness, which can bring depression with it, either as a consequence of living with illness or, indeed, as a feature of the illness itself: inflammatory and autoimmune diseases can affect the brain, causing neuropsychiatric disease along with other symptoms. The trouble was that in the face of uncertainty, this doctor viewed my problems as exclusively psychological.

Meanwhile, things were getting worse: it was increasingly hard to remember words and details. Teaching my poetry workshop, I found myself talking to the students about "the season that comes after winter, when flowers grow." Yet some part of me thought that perhaps this was what everyone in her midthirties felt. Pain, exhaustion, a leaden mind.

That November, I calculated the time it was taking me to manage my health care. By now, I had nine doctors—a GP, an endocrinologist, a rheumatologist, a neurologist, a dermatologist, an ob-gyn, a sports medicine doctor (who specialized in hip and knee injuries), a nutritionist, and a reproductive endocrinologist, to help with trying to get pregnant.

Because I'd begun having severe headaches while traveling in Texas, a clinician there had ordered an MRI of my brain, which showed a lesion, and my GP and neurologist wanted to have a look at the scan because of the numbness and electric shocks I was experiencing. It took five phone calls and several faxes to get my records. (Faxes? I had to walk to a copy shop a mile away to be able to send such a thing.) And it was never easy to get an appointment with a new specialist: each time I saw a doctor who suggested I see a different specialist, I had to resign myself to waiting four to six weeks.

Often one of these new doctors needed or requested information that the other doctors had, and I would spend hours speaking to medical-records departments, printing out forms that authorized sharing my information, faxing them to the doctor's office, then calling to confirm the receipt of that fax. Even when forms were electronic—most were, even then—the doctors' offices typically didn't want the information being emailed. The overburdened administrators usually sounded annoyed at having to deal with more paperwork and would snap that it was impossible to send the records before my appointment with Dr. So-and-so—who then would not have the necessary information on hand when I saw him and would ask me to come back for a follow-up.

God forbid *I* wanted a copy of my lab reports and had forgotten to ask; it took hounding and harassing to get them. More than one office informed me that it could take three weeks to transfer records. This in a world where I can order a life-sized Bigfoot statue from Amazon and have it delivered to my doorstep overnight. Some doctors flat-out told me they didn't want me to have copies of my lab results because I would "make myself worried" or "get confused."

During these months, I calculated, I spent a day and a half per month just moving paper and electronic records from doctor to doctor. I spent an additional three days traveling to doctors' appointments, during which I often waited for an hour or more to be seen for ten minutes. (Or fifteen, when my doctor had time.) Putting it all together, I realized that each month I was losing close to five out of twenty workdays—nearly a quarter of my work time.

The bigger problem, though, is that all these hoops made it much more likely that I would just give up or fail to follow through. At times I did. When I later asked Jack Cochran, the former executive director of the Permanente Federation, what happens to patients who don't have the energy or the means to persevere in connecting their disconnected doctors, he said, "They fall through the cracks, and they suffer in their own world, alone."

THINGS ON THE MEDICAL-RECORDS FRONT, at least, are better now. The 21st Century Cures Act—which went into full effect in April 2021—mandated that patients have the right to access their records and doctors' notes electronically, and usually all one has to do is sign up for a MyChart account to get those notes. But the system as a whole remains ill-equipped to deal with chronic illness. It's technologically proficient but emotionally deficient, much better at treating acute problems than chronic ones: for every instance of expert treatment, skilled surgery, or innovative problem-solving, there are countless cases of substandard care, overlooked diagnoses, bureaucratic bungling, and even outright antagonism between doctor and patient.

Even before I got really sick, I had spent a lot of time in doctors' offices and hospitals, due to a succession of gynecological surgeries and trips to specialists for MRIs, and because I was in and out of doctors' offices and hospitals with my mother while she was being treated for cancer. I was impressed by how precise surgery had become. (The first time I had surgery for endometriosis, an ovarian cyst the size of a grapefruit was removed via a tiny incision. I was running again within five days.) I was struck, too, by the kindness of many of my mother's nurses and physicians. But I was also startled by the profound discomfort I felt, especially in hospitals. Doctors at times seemed brusque and even hostile toward us. The lighting was harsh, the food terrible, the rooms loud and devoid of comfort. Weren't people there to heal? This did not appear to matter. What mattered was the whole bureaucratic apparatus of "care": the beeping monitors and hourly check-ins and forced wakings, the elaborate (and frequently futile) interventions painstakingly performed on the terminally ill. At the hospital, I always felt like Alice at the Mad Hatter's tea party: I had woken up in a world that seemed utterly logical to its inhabitants but quite mad to me.

In America's techno-medical system, a person who is sick becomes something less than a person on entering a doctor's office. As early as the turn of the twentieth century, critics had begun to complain that patients were now "numbers on charts, shadows on x-ray plates, and smears on slides," notes the medical historian Charles Rosenberg. Things only got worse as technological advances and corporatization transformed the American medical system into one characterized by silos and high-tech specialization, resulting in a bureaucratic remove from the patient. "Any patient in a hospital, when we take their clothes away and lay them in a bed, starts to lose identity; after a few days, they all start to merge into a single passive body," writes Terrence Holt, a geriatric specialist at the University of North Carolina at Chapel Hill.

My mother and I were among the luckier ones, as relatively privileged white women. My mother received prompt, attentive care (though male doctors often felt a need to comment patronizingly on her weight to me, as if I would share their sentiments). Although I encountered doctors who dismissed me, I had the means to keep searching for the caring physicians who would eventually become partners in my quest for health. But those who cannot afford (financially or energetically) to keep searching sometimes stop, stuck in the trap of unidentified illness. Class, race, language—these can all be barriers to good care. Overt racism and unconscious bias toward people of color, women, and transgender patients is rampant in some hospitals and practices, where health care workers—according to many doctors' own accounts—routinely refer, to choose just two well-documented examples, to obese people as "beached whales" or to Latinx patients as having "Hispanic hysterical syndrome." A 2018 study found that only 85 percent of doctors surveyed were willing to provide routine care to transgender patients, while a recent survey of transgender and non-binary people found that 19 percent "reported being refused care outright because they were transgender or gender non-conforming." For Black people, everyday tensions are backed by a long history of medical apartheid, epitomized in the decades-long Tuskegee experiment, in which physicians identified Black patients with syphilis and then withheld the penicillin treatment that would have cured them in order to study the full course of the infection. No wonder many patients distrust doctors.

Even as a white cisgender woman, I faced indifference and incuriosity. For example, although I had grown up hiking and camping in the Northeast, for years no doctor asked if I had been tested for Lyme disease or other tick-borne illnesses. None except for Dr. E tried to ascertain if there was a history of autoimmune disease in my family. Writing these words ten years later, I am astonished by these facts, but I know from interviewing patients and talking to friends that I was hardly alone. The pattern is this: A patient goes to the doctor to explain that something seems very wrong. When tests turn nothing up, the patient is told she is fine, and emerges without answers, questioning everything she thought she knew about her body and her perceptions. I grew practiced in choosing only a few symptoms to tell my doctors about, and I didn't mention the many other doctors I had seen: physicians often assume patients who "doctor shop" are problem patients. I also quickly learned one of the worst things I could do was to show up prepared with prior medical records. A 1988 paper by T. C. O'Dowd coined the term "heartsink patients" to describe patients who "exasperate, defeat, and overwhelm" their doctors. I didn't want to be such a patient—a patient who seems to ask too much.

The problem stems in part from the challenges bureaucracy poses to doctor-patient relationships: How can well-intentioned doctors listen openly to the woes of chronically ill patients when they themselves are frustrated and burned out? Often my doctors, bogged down in paperwork, were working at what the cardiologist Sandeep Jauhar calls "hyperspeed" in *Doctored: The Disillusionment of an American Physician*; nearly always they were running behind schedule and apologetic. To their credit, they never implied that I was crazy, or seeking attention, though I have interviewed many people who were told as much by their doctors. But few of the physicians I saw seemed to believe that anything was significantly wrong.

And so, as I trudged from specialist to specialist in the fall and winter of 2012, getting enough blood drawn to satisfy a thirsty vampire, I blamed myself. I felt responsible for the fact that I didn't know how to speak to the doctors with the words that would get them, as I thought of it, "on my side." I steeled myself before appointments, yet I never managed to ask even half of my questions without feeling that I'd already imposed and exhausted the physician's generosity. "To speak our life as we feel it is a freedom we mostly choose not to take," the writer Deborah Levy notes. Now, when I needed to exercise this freedom, I couldn't figure out how to do so, so accustomed—acculturated—was I to taking my cues from what others wanted to hear. Often my physicians interrupted me just as I'd begun to talk. (Doctors tend to interrupt patients after eleven seconds of speech.)

One unseasonably mild day, I left a new doctor's office in Manhattan, sweating under my silk shirt, and leaned woozily against a dirty Prius, breathless with hurt. Her office was busy, and she had patronized me and rushed me out the door. I felt more acutely alone than ever. I had no ally—worse, the encounter left me with a rusty taste in my mouth, a sense that perhaps I didn't deserve an ally. For this is the strange thing about a vulnerability that remains unseen by others, an illness that is unacknowledged by society. It is the *sick person* whose worldview warps, the wounded one who absorbs the idea that the most indelible aspect of her present condition is in fact a defect, a distortion of her own making.

CONTEMPORARY MEDICINE prides itself on patient-centered care, but it is startlingly inattentive—even actively indifferent—to patients' emotional needs. For patients with chronic illness, with its upheaval of life, this indifference poses a particular challenge. In chronic illness, the patient does not have a problem that can be solved quickly but a disease to be managed, physically and psychologically. Such illnesses can be intractable, messy, mysterious. And doctors don't like to manage; they like to *fix*. Medical education emphasizes *solutions* and is often "equated with cure," according to a 2005 study of doctor-patient relationships in chronic illness. Unfortunately, "the treatment of chronic disease conflicts so fundamentally with these expectations that it tends to be neglected." Indeed, a 2004 Johns Hopkins study found that nearly two thirds of doctors surveyed felt inadequately trained in key aspects of care of the chronically ill.

Doctors prefer acute care, David Cutler, a Harvard economist who specializes in health care reform, told me, because it is easier to work with a patient in a mechanistic way, to anesthetize someone, say, in order to fix a broken bone. (An anesthetized patient is also a quiet patient, he pointed out.) Chronic illness requires doctors to work with patients on behavioral modifications—slow, frustrating work. "It's very hard to get people to change their behaviors in any way—working with people is the hardest thing," Cutler said. "The best kind of patient for this purpose," the psychiatrist T. F. Main wrote, "is one who from great suffering and danger of life or sanity responds quickly to a treatment that interests his doctor and thereafter remains completely well." The patient diagnosed with Lyme disease whose symptoms fail to go away after a course of antibiotics, the patient with medically unexplained pain—these are precisely the opposite kind of patient.

The problem isn't doctors so much as the system, in short. Today, the typical medical appointment is fifteen minutes long, which is not enough time for patients with a complex condition to go over symptoms and ask questions, or for a doctor to coach a patient through lifestyle changes. The short appointments have a history: rising costs in the 1970s were the catalyst for "managed care"—basically, our current system, in which insurance companies like Aetna and UnitedHealthcare negotiate with networks of doctors to determine how much care patients get, whom we can see, for how long, and at what price. To rein in costs, insurance companies have set fees lower and lower, and doctors work faster and faster, especially when they are in large medical networks that require them to cram in a set number of visits per day.

Compounding all these issues, health care is divided into silos, with each specialist operating individually, keeping their own records, and referring patients who need to see other specialists to their own favored doctors. The model works especially poorly for autoimmunity and other chronic illnesses: no one is in charge of coordinating care. Silos fail to support "the whole patient," an editorial from the Foundation of the American College of Healthcare Executives notes; there are communication gaps. "Deep silo–based specialists don't always work well together," Jack Cochran told me. "And who's in the middle? The patient, not the doctor." The Affordable Care Act aimed to fix this by incentivizing coordination of care, penalizing hospitals for excessive readmission of patients (which would indicate that hospitals are not getting to the root cause of their patients' problems), but these incentives barely made a dent in the superstructure of modern American medicine. Then, too, health care in the United States operates predominantly on a fee-for-service basis, which rewards doctors for doing as many procedures and ordering as many tests as possible rather than for offering the best *care* possible.

The bureaucracy frustrates doctors and patients both. And it places an added burden on those for whom the costs and complexities of navigating a fragmented system are a barrier to access. Given these systemic realities, it comes as no surprise that health care outcomes in the United States correlate to income levels. "The greater one's income, the lower one's likelihood of disease and premature death," a 2015 report on health care equity from the Urban Institute and the Center on Society and Health at Virginia Commonwealth University found. Those who cannot afford health insurance or doctors' copayments are less likely to seek care or to navigate a complicated system that shuttles them from doctor to doctor, racking up fees as they go.

Health care outcomes also vary according to race. A 2020 editorial in *The Lancet* stated bluntly, "Racism is a public health emergency of global concern. It is the root cause of continued disparities in death and disease between Black and white people in the USA." For a complex array of reasons including structural racism and deep-rooted bias in medicine, patients of color don't get the care they need.

As a result, the United States is in the midst of a crisis rooted not just in rising costs but in the very meaning and ethics of care. It is difficult to be a patient for long without coming up against the hard truth that what you are searching for and what your doctor is offering are two entirely different things. One of the underacknowledged facts of being ill is how difficult and saddening the encounters with the medical system can be. The situation is so extreme—the impasse so obvious—that at Davos in 2014, Mark Bertolini, the CEO of Aetna, speaking of his own experiences guiding his sixteen-year-old son through the health care system, exclaimed, "The patient really isn't a person. The patient is a diagnosis. The patient is that day's crisis." He continued: "That focus on disease rather than the individual doesn't create advocacy for the person or coordination of the care. My role became the coordinator of the care."

"I want to be treated as a person, but I'm only a patient to them," I said to Jim one chilly winter night, when streaks of clouds gauzily wrapped a full moon outside our kitchen window, after another appointment. I was almost brokenhearted. I had gone in hoping for help. Instead, the doctor had shrugged when I asked if he could help me: "We're *all* tired, Meghan."

"Our system is great if you need surgery," I said to Jim, through tears I fought back. "But when you are suffering day in and out, it feels terrible to go to the doctor's office and barely be spoken to." We were sitting at our table, the radiator steaming and clanking, plates of takeout Mediterranean food in front of us. We had made a home. I had a good job and wonderful friends. If I had not been sick, I would have felt I was, at thirty-six, in the prime of my life, doing work I wanted to do, ready to start a family, past the worst of my grief at the early loss of my mother. Instead, I floated in uncertainty. Jim looked at me, the overhead light shadowing his jaw, his eyes grave. "I know," he said, and although he didn't say more, I could feel futility weighing on him like one of the too-heavy bags he packed whenever we traveled.

. . .

THE MOST ALARMING FACT I learned, when I began my research, was how quickly doctors' empathy wanes. Multiple studies show that it plunges in the third year of medical school, declining when students start seeing patients on rotation and, overworked and overtired, they realize that there is too much work to be done in too little time, or end up distancing themselves self-protectively from their patients in order to survive.

Then, too, doctors may have little understanding of the recognition their chronically ill patients want from them. Arthur Frank, a medical sociologist, points out that the ill are busy trying to formulate a story to help them navigate their new identity. Being ill, after all, is unwelcome, foreign, confusing. It interrupts your plans for the present and, when you are chronically ill, for your future. But at first very little is clear to the patient, and that lack of understanding—of control—is terrifying. And so the patient invests time and effort trying to figure out a new story; she wants someone to help write that new story by making space for the loss that has occurred, the harm done, and by seeing it as the unique loss it is. In a treatment setting, then, patients want to be *listened* to, not least because they view doctors as authorities conferring further meaning and recognition, which doctors may not realize. One young woman I interviewed noted, "The emotional journey has been as hard as the physical one. The fear I feel, in combination with busy doctors who don't have time to listen, has really affected me."

Being heard by your doctor isn't just an emotional need but a physical one: patients benefit clinically from feeling cared for. The emotional and the physical, science is learning, are more intertwined than we once understood. Many studies have suggested that emotional care—interpersonal warmth—has a measurable effect on patients' outcomes. For example, the incidence of severe diabetes complications in patients of doctors who rate high on a standard empathy scale is a remarkable

40 percent lower than in patients whose doctors do poorly on the empathy scale, Danielle Ofri, an internist at New York's Bellevue Hospital, reports in *What Doctors Feel*. "This is comparable," she points out, "to the benefits seen with the most intensive medical therapy for diabetes."

In a study of placebo effects conducted by Ted Kaptchuk at Harvard, patients with irritable bowel syndrome were told they were taking part in a study about the benefits of acupuncture. Two groups were treated with "sham" acupuncture. One group received treatment from practitioners who had only perfunctory interactions with the patients, stating brusquely that they "knew what to do." The second group received treatment from a researcher who warmly asked questions about them and expressed empathy for their suffering. The group treated by the empathetic researcher had more symptom reduction than the group treated by the brusque researcher. In fact, the percentage of patients in the "empathetic" group reporting adequate relief in symptoms was as high as that reported in clinical trials of drugs typically used in IBS.

"What Kaptchuk demonstrated is what some medical thinkers have begun to call the 'care effect,'" Nathanael Johnson wrote in *Wired* in 2013, "the idea that the opportunity for patients to feel heard and cared for can improve their health."

In other words, the effects of empathy are real, and they are measurable. A 2002 *New England Journal of Medicine* study even found that a placebo treatment worked as well as arthroscopic surgery for patients with arthritis of the knee. (At the time, 650,000 such operations were being performed a year.) Orthopedic surgeons complained about the study's findings, insisting that their patients felt better after surgery. The patients who had been operated on did feel better. But so did the patients who received a caring nonsurgical "treatment."

THE RISE OF PATIENTS' RIGHTS in the 1970s and 1980s was supposed to change all this, leading to a more collaborative relationship between patient and doctor, based on informed consent. But the balance of power is still tilted in favor of the doctor. When a patient tries to talk to a rushed doctor, wanting both assistance and agency, the conversation is often fraught on both sides.

Doctors still label patients who refuse to take their medications "non-compliant" regardless of whether the patients have good reasons for doing so—for example, antiseizure medication can make an epilepsy patient too groggy to function at work. My mother, when she had colorectal cancer, was said by a doctor to have "failed" chemotherapy when her disease progressed. Wasn't it the other way around? Medicine has been trying to reform such uses of language (more often now, it speaks of "treatment failure" and "nonadherent" patients), but in a quick Google search one morning I found the following headline: "Treatment Options of Patients with Chronic Hepatitis C Who Have Failed Prior Therapy."

This language of patient blaming is not accidental. One can imagine the special helplessness that physicians must often feel, the tragedies witnessed that must be quickly filed away. A doctor's job, like a gambler's, is intimately tied up with failure; the house always wins over time. That significance is what some doctors avoid grappling with. "One of the most venerable psychological self-defense stratagems is to erect protective barriers between oneself and one's patients," the radiologist Richard Gunderman writes in a report on patient blaming. "These habits of speech contribute to a presumption that the responsibility for failure lies with the patient." By making the patient the problem, clinicians at least still have faith in their own ability to help.

Jack Cochran thinks that medicine needs to reevaluate the doctor-patient relationship. "We call it the doctor-patient relationship, but in many ways it's the doctor-down-to-the-patient relationship," he told me. "Patients need to be relentlessly assertive and ask their questions as many times as necessary, until they get answers they can understand. It is their body; it is their well-being; they deserve an answer. It is up to the doctors then to say, 'I know it's this,' or 'I don't know, but I'll try to learn more,' or 'I am stumped and think we should get additional input.'"

In 2015, I met with Cochran, and I asked him why it was that doctors so often dismissed patients with vague symptoms.

"The reason is this—you're coming to me, and my stock-in-trade is expertise. You're coming to me because I have this brain full of stuff that you need. But if my brain can't do what it needs to do, then I'm a fraud, or a flawed doctor, or inadequate, or stupid, and that ain't easy on me, because I've always made A's in chemistry, I've always passed my boards, I've always been high on the food chain of knowledge acquisition and management. It doesn't feel good to me, to be mortal. I'm failing you—*I'm* a failure."

Susan Block, the Harvard professor and palliative care pioneer I had spoken to, told me something similar when I asked her why she thought doctors tended to dismiss patients with unclear lab results—why they so often decided, as she had put it, that the patient was "cuckoo."

"I think it has to do with physicians' difficulties in tolerating uncertainty," she told me. "The nagging worry is that if you can't see it objectively, you are missing something medically or being bamboozled somehow—fooled by the patient. That is scary to doctors. A lot of the dysfunctional behavior toward people with the more ambiguous chronic illnesses stems from the fact that the doctor gets anxious about either missing something medical or being made a fool of by a patient who is psychiatrically ill. That kind of mistake feels humiliating; an effort to avoid it takes the form of pathologizing or labeling the patient 'psychologically ill.'"

To be sure, the patient, unlike the customer, can't always be right, and good care demands that doctors be honest about what they do and don't see, as well as the potential harms of treatment. I found myself thinking about how hard I would have found it to recommend next steps for me, were I my own physicians. They had no way to know how sick I really was, when my labs didn't show it and I looked OK. This is why the doctors who took the time to acknowledge that they could see I was sick for reasons they didn't understand made a powerful impact on me, far beyond what they imagined, I am sure. Their words were like a rope thrown across a frightening abyss.

IN 1926, DR. FRANCIS W. PEABODY instructed Harvard medical students, "The secret of the care of the patient is in caring for the patient." To most of us, the body seems strangely—perhaps terrifyingly—solitary when it is sick. But the sick body is always in dialogue with others. Even at the moment it seems most isolated the body remains "dyadic," as the sociologist Arthur Frank puts it: in dialogue with the medical system, with spouses, and so on. Research like Kaptchuk's underscores the material and corporeal reality of Frank's point: the body is a site of social encounter, not a vessel for American hyperindividualism.

The questions raised by this fresh understanding of the dyadic nature of illness are significant. Should patients have a larger role in shaping the health care system? Does the "care" part of health care matter in any material way—should our system do more to recognize how much time a doctor spends on this intangible work? Does America's broken health care system require rethinking not just economically but ethically? Does medicine matter as a moral enterprise? Both patients and many doctors would answer yes, yes, yes, and yes. During our conversation, I asked Susan Block if it was reasonable for chronically ill patients to want an emotionally supportive relationship with their doctors. "Absolutely," she said. "If we can't do that, we really are practicing only half of what medicine is and can be."

Soon after I began writing this book, I attended a talk about patients' rights at Harvard Medical School on a cloudy afternoon punctuated by snow flurries. I was surprised to hear various people high in administrative hospital practice talking about their work "overseeing" the patient and speaking generally of patients as if they were irrational, dim-witted children who couldn't be trusted to make their own decisions. These *were* the people who thought care was important, people who had trundled out in the freezing cold to listen to ideas about what they could be doing better for their patients. And yet years of thinking about patients in terms of their compliance had given them a dismissive attitude toward the very people they sought to help.

In pain, exhausted, and angry, I, too, was swept up in futile pageantry. I signed up for appointments, I waited, I got my hopes up, I went and sat in shoddy, sad offices with pictures of sailboats on the wall and greasily thumbed magazines on side tables sourced from bulk office furniture suppliers. The actual encounter was always confusing, eleven minutes of liminal contact in which I tried to conduct myself in a way that would make the doctor like me, in the hope they would take some true interest in my plight. But their day was full of tests to order, bureaucracy to cut through, an education that taught them not to say, "I don't know what's wrong with you." And so we stood together in a tiny, antiseptic room, the doctor and the patient, a world apart.

SIX

ALTERNATIVES

Alternative medicine appeals to many chronically ill people precisely because it offers what its name suggests: an alternative to a vast, bureaucratic, impersonal medical system that leaves little room for the personal side of sickness. "To the extent that modern physicalist medicine does offer any kind of story about illness," the historian Anne Harrington writes in *The Cure Within: A History of Mind-Body Medicine,* "it is a story that is as impersonal as they come: it is all about the disease rather than the patient, and it is articulated using a specialized vocabulary of tissue, blood, and biochemistry." In the face of persistent pain or a recalcitrant illness, people confronted with a mechanistic or partial explanation "long for something better—a better story." Certainly I did.

Alternative medicine is built around the twin rituals of offering soothing care and focused attention. What exhausted, chronically ill person couldn't use a supplement, or an authority figure asking how their spirits are, suggesting stress relief, offering plain old recognition and comfort? "You're not crazy, and yes, you *can* feel better."

It should come as no surprise that alternative medicine rose to new heights of popularity in the 1990s, as Western medicine became more technocratic. A 2016 NIH survey found that Americans were spending $30.2 billion a year on alternative and complementary medicine. The desire for *care* is one reason so many people turn to it. "What the language of alternative medicine understands is that when we feel bad we want something unambiguously good," the writer Eula Biss aptly notes in *On Immunity: An Inoculation*. In this case, I wanted the unambiguously good all the more because I felt ambiguously bad.

Steeped in the Western tradition, I initially distrusted integrative doctors and alternative practitioners, even as I consulted them. I still saw my Western specialists as authorities, and there was a lot of unscientific (and disproved) information shared online in the name of alternative medicine. I found it hard to know what to trust or how to differentiate what was at the cutting edge from what was known to be false. But as more and more "small things" went wrong—endometriosis, hives, the labral tear in my hip, the arthritis in my neck, the thyroid disease, the failure to get pregnant, the fatigue and brain fog—I had started to see my body differently, not as a collection of parts but as an entangled system. And this realization catalyzed a radical change not just in how I experienced my health but also in how I saw the medical system and the road to getting the care that I needed.

After I caught Jim googling "symptoms of leukemia," I decided to see a New York integrative doctor whom several acquaintances had recommended—I'll call him Dr. K. My friends warned me that he was very expensive: a single consultation would set me back five hundred dollars, and like most so-called integrative doctors, he did not take insurance, for similar reasons that some top-tier Western doctors did not: the bureaucracy involved made it hard to spend longer amounts of time with patients. I did not have a spare five hundred dollars, but I had a credit card, and my insurance at the time reimbursed me for 80 percent of the cost of out-of-network visits.

Many practitioners of alternative medicine are "naturopaths" who have attended a four-year accredited graduate degree program, which follows some of the traditional medical curriculum and then branches off to teach holistic and whole-body approaches to health. But there is a growing world of "integrative" and "functional" doctors: MDs who use Western medicine along with alternative practices. Usually, they aim to treat the patient as a whole person, seeking to unearth the complex root causes of an illness rather than offer a quick local fix. Integrative and functional medicine also aim to treat the body *before* it becomes pathologically ill, supporting it by instituting practices of self-care around nutrition, sleep, and stress, restoring the body to higher function, as it were. Where conventional medicine focuses on fixing, integrative medicine focuses on healing and prevention.

Typically, a first appointment with an alternative or integrative practitioner lasts an hour, during which the doctor or practitioner goes over many aspects of the patient's life. The patient fills out a long intake form, which may include questions about sleep, anxiety, caffeine consumption, what you typically eat for breakfast, lunch, and dinner, whether you're in a supportive relationship, whether you have "spots of pain" or feelings of being faint or cold, for example. Often, it asks patients to rate their stress level on a scale of one to ten, and sometimes to identify its sources (work, relationships, and so on).

In my experience, filling out that form is the first step in a ritual: already the patient feels *paid attention to*, which brings with it a certain feeling of calm security, as if the practitioner were a surrogate parent, benevolently observing your every action, urging you on to a better life and a more realized self. This sense of being paid attention to—the conversation that happens between practitioner and patient—is key to alternative medicine's popularity and even its successes. Alternative medicine also involves a strong element of touch, which is neglected in Western medicine. For example, an acupuncturist takes your pulse and looks at your tongue, your skin, maybe your eyes. The act of placing needles becomes a kind of care, after which you are left to relax, with soothing music and candles, in a womb-like room. I remember being amazed that my private aches and pains, invisible to my medical doctors, were quickly found by my massage therapists and acupuncturists and addressed without my even having to point them out. Such low-key, soothing attention is, to put it plainly, *nice*.

On the day of my appointment with Dr. K, I headed downtown to his office. It had a spare, bright, Scandinavian vibe. Instead of the fluorescent lights and synthetic seating of the typical doctor's office, it boasted natural light from high windows, a midcentury modern couch, and a coffee table scattered with books about interior decorating.

Dr. K met with me right away, smiling broadly as he shook my hand. A small, friendly man with bright eyes, he exuded a warm calm. He was an advocate of detoxification and his own skin seemed to glow in testimony to its benefits.

"So, what brings you here?" he asked, leaning toward me.

I explained that I'd been suffering from mysterious fatigue and brain fog, as well as pain and other amorphous symptoms. I just didn't feel *right*. He did an exam; I'd brought my medical records, and he looked carefully through them.

"Whatever else is going on," he said, "it looks like you're run-down by exhaustion and by viruses. I see here that you tested positive some months back for active Epstein-Barr, CMV, and parvovirus. Today, we will do blood work to see what, exactly, we can figure out." He suggested I needed to work on restoring my body's own resources using an herbal antiviral regime and a series of IV vitamin drips (known as "Myers's cocktails") to raise the level of nutrients in my body, helping it perform better. He gave me herbs called "adaptogens," which are supposed to help the body adapt to stress, and offered me another salivary cortisol test to see if my cortisol production was out of whack (leading to fatigue), then led me back to the infusion room. Two years earlier, I'd seen people getting these drips, sitting in oversized leather chairs that resembled Barcaloungers, at the office of another doctor I'd visited. The whole thing had seemed creepy. Today, I was desperate to try one as soon as possible. In the night world of illness, the prospect of a vitamin cocktail is a real thrill.

I left with a few hundred dollars' worth of supplements and waited for my test results to come back. A few weeks later, on my second visit, Dr. K told me I had—once again—high levels of active viral antibodies, this time for Epstein-Barr virus and CMV. I had also tested positive for significant amounts of heavy metals in my blood—including mercury and lead, which many people on the illness forums I frequented talked about, as well as a remarkably high amount of thallium, a metal used in industrial products, which was a less common finding. As a result, Dr. K suggested I consider something called "chelation therapy," where a synthetic amino acid is injected into the body to help draw heavy metals out of the tissues.

Whether such extraction is beneficial for a wide variety of patients is still not entirely clear, and conventional doctors think that chelation may harm some patients, especially when conducted more than once. To Western doctors, chelation is an example of alternative medicine's dangerous embrace of non-evidence-based treatment in the dubious name of cleansing. It can cause liver damage and kidney problems. Some evidence exists that it simply moves the heavy metals around the body without stripping it of them. A study of toddlers with high lead levels who were treated by chelation failed to find any neuro-behavioral benefits, though this hardly seemed to settle the question. But a 2013 study found that patients over fifty treated with chelation therapy experienced a drop of 18 percent in cardiovascular events. Eric Topol, a prominent cardiologist, told *The New York Times* that conventional medicine should take note of the study, which "does appear to signal a benefit. That challenges the prevailing dogma."

When you feel ambiguously bad, the idea of a drip that will slowly strip your body of an unnatural accretion of toxins and other detritus of living is a powerful one. Like many people I had met online, I had begun to internalize the notion that a toxic modernity was afflicting me, contaminating my body. A ritualistic purging of that modern contamination (even by way of a distinctively modern treatment) appealed to me. It suggested the possibility of undoing what society had wrought. Once you've been told you have toxic metal in your body, you want to get it out. People I knew had found it helpful, and Dr. K told me he had seen it benefit his patients. Then he warned me that the process would make me smell of garlic to other people, though I wouldn't be able to smell it myself. "You will want to plan to go straight home afterward," he said, with a wry smile.

On the day I went for my chelation, a few women and one man sat in their oversized leather loungers. One woman gave a little cry of pain when the nurse pricked her with the thick IV needle. I sat back. The cocktail dripping into my veins produced a metallic taste in my mouth. Sometimes it felt quite cold going in my vein, and my elbow and upper arm began to ache, an ache as deep as heartsickness.

After sitting in my Barcalounger for three hours, until the drip was done flushing through my veins, I headed home on the subway, exhausted. Inside, Jim reached to kiss me and then gave me a puzzled look. "You smell weird," he said.

I couldn't smell a thing.

As he wrinkled his nose at me, it struck me: this situation was the exact inverse of my experience of being sick, in which *I* could detect that something was wrong, but no one else could.

THE DISCOURSE OF NATURAL MEDICINE—of alternative and integrative medicine, of wellness culture—draws on our nostalgia for an imagined past. It is a discourse not only of optimization but of regret, though this aspect is rarely acknowledged: regret that we cannot undo what we have done to the polluted world; that we cannot have the best of science without having the worst of it; that we live atomized, exhausted, late-capitalist lives, running from here to there, eyes on our phones. The "natural approach" appeals because it trades on notions of purity as a way of restoring health. It promises to return us to a time when our bodies were untainted by modernity, technology, and pollution, a path to a prelapsarian physical self, capable of almost anything, including self-healing. In this view, implicitly, illness is almost a deviation from the natural: a problem we can control through obsessive self-care. There is at the core of alternative medicine a strangely utopian notion of health, a belief that traditional medicine is itself toxic and the body is a healing machine that tends toward health, as opposed to a system prone to glitches and major dysfunction that only technological and pharmaceutical intervention can help—a body that dies. Medicated and ill, I wanted to reach that past—or, I corrected myself, I wanted to strip the present of the invisible contaminants that might be making me sick without my knowing it. I wanted the best of everything.

Of course, while this nostalgia contains real truths about our contemporary life, it elides truth about life before the advent of modern medicine. Our nostalgia—be it for "natural" immunity resulting from contracting an infection, or for the nourishment of raw milk, or just for the purity of preindustrial life—leaves out of its vision the high death rate from infections, the dirty water that spread typhoid, the rancid unpasteurized milk that sometimes killed babies, and the basic struggle to survive. It leaves out our longer lives and our lower rates of infant and maternal mortality. Americans' embrace of the "natural approach" is a rebuke to the dominant social structures of our time—Big Pharma, Big Medicine, Big Tech. But in a crucial way it is also in thrall to one of the most powerful contemporary Western delusions: namely, the idea that we can control the outcomes of our lives, in this case through self-purification.

This was a delusion I was still entirely in the grips of. There was a spiritual aspect to my performance of self-care. I was trying, through ritual, to heal my broken life, to find continuity again.

BUT ON A MORE PRACTICAL LEVEL, I had come to believe that I was most likely to get answers from an integrative doctor with an open-minded approach to healing. While I had great faith in science, I had begun to see that I stood at the edge of what medicine knew, and that medicine, given its own conservative, data-driven, evidence-based approach, had run out of things to offer me. I needed something else: I needed help getting through my day, and help figuring out why I felt better on some days than on others. Alternative and functional medicine's attention to nutrition and sleep and improving my health around the edges had a great deal to offer me, even if it was just the alleviation or improvement of my worst symptoms, or a few more days of energy and focus. "I need a disease detective," I told Jim one night, something that ten-minute appointments did not allow even my most caring physicians to be. Integrative doctors had that kind of time; they were set up to listen in detail to patients, and they believed in intervening to improve function in the interconnected systems of the body. They saw my symptoms not as individual problems in separate organs but as related manifestations of a system under physical stress of some kind.

The integrative doctors I saw—I tried a few different ones—found some anomalies in my lab work. I had a positive ANA result (again, autoantibodies to cell DNA), which could indicate an autoimmune connective tissue disease similar to lupus. My magnesium was low, my vitamin D was low, and my ferritin (a storage form of iron) was almost nonexistent. My blood pressure sometimes dropped to 82/49. All this, Dr. K said, could be the result of an infection. In addition, I had two polymorphisms in the MTHFR gene—the "motherfucker gene," as online patients called it—which meant that my body didn't process folic acid and B_{12} as effectively as it should, potentially leading to fatigue and neurological problems. The many food sensitivities suggested that I also had what was called "leaky gut"—intestinal permeability—and less than optimal function in my hypothalamic-pituitary-adrenal axis. This could be contributing to low levels of "adrenal fatigue."

When I asked a conventional medical doctor what she thought of this approach, she told me that from her perspective the findings were nonspecific and that Western medicine didn't recognize adrenal fatigue as a reality, since some studies found no significant differences between controls and patients with fatigue. Even so, she said, medicine *did* recognize a form of adrenal insufficiency known as "Addison's disease," in which the adrenal glands produce too little cortisol and aldosterone. She offered to test my cortisol to make sure that wasn't the case. Here in a nutshell was the difference: one system looks for small variations from a pattern and aims to remedy them with herbs and lifestyle management that (it says) will prevent more serious disease, the other looks for an extreme deviation in adrenal hormone levels that manifests in profound illness, and treats it with powerful steroids, but regards minor deviations as outside its purview. Where the evidence stops, the doctors' hands are tied. Or rather, when you live outside the boundaries of known pathology, conventional medicine hesitates to intervene. The positive ANA that my integrative doctors took seriously was seen as not yet meaningful by some of my conventional doctors, in the absence of other findings; many people had positive ANAs without being sick. (One physician failed to even tell me I had a positive ANA test, I realized years later, looking at my labs.) I deeply respected their evidence-based approach, but I also knew I was not healthy.

Still, faced with two opposing narratives I struggled: What *did* these results mean? Were they real cause for alarm, or were my integrative doctors looking for problems, as a friend of mine worried they were, to charge me hundreds of dollars for supplements? The latter question would have concerned me more if I had felt great and these practitioners were telling me I was sick. But I felt as though I might be dying. I was therefore grateful for the integrative doctors' willingness to intervene "around the edges," as one put it, and to act on clues that might lead us to treatments, if not answers. Dr. K nudged me to meditate and sleep more; another integrative doctor realized I was reacting badly to eggs, and persuaded me to stop eating them. The adjustments such doctors encouraged me to make—their willingness to work with me on lifestyle changes—helped me.

Even with insurance covering out-of-network care, the costs of seeing integrative doctors were still significant—the year I met with Dr. K, I spent, before reimbursement, about twenty-two thousand dollars on appointments, medical treatment such as IVs, lab work, and supplements. I rotated my portion of the costs on 0 percent APR credit cards, betting that I would get well enough to make the money to pay them off.

I did the Myers's cocktails every few weeks; they helped tremendously, for whatever reason. (My brain fog lifted for a few days.) I was given—or told to buy, really—hundreds of dollars' worth of supplements. I had food sensitivity testing that indicated I was sensitive to wheat, barley, eggs, beef, dairy, pork, sesame, cranberries, and corn—my body, according to the tests, was mounting a delayed immune response to those foods. Western medicine doesn't put much stock in food sensitivity tests, which measure not the IgE antibodies that cause food allergies—immediate immune reactions—but the IgG, IgA, and IgM antibodies that may create a slower inflammatory response to a given food. Because I was not sure what to make of the testing, I got allergy testing from two doctors who sent my blood to different labs. Identical results came back. I had already stopped eating gluten and eggs, which I knew made me feel bad. Now I also gave up cranberry, sesame, dairy, beef, and corn—none of which, to my knowledge, had ever made me feel bad. At the instruction of a doctor who noted that I was seriously allergic to dust mites, I washed my sheets and pillows twice a week in hot water. I went to bed by nine p.m. I never wavered in my total commitment to health. (If this is exhausting to read, imagine what it was like to live through.) As the treatments with Dr. K went on, the fatigue, the deadly enervation, lifted enough to help me function better.

I couldn't figure out where that sky-high thallium level had come from, though. Then, one day *Mother Jones* ran a story about kale, which I ate twice every day in my attempts to detoxify my liver and stick to a blood-sugar-balancing Paleo diet. It was one of my "safe" foods. But the leafy green vegetable that had come to symbolize artisanal hipster health is uniquely adept, some research suggests, at drawing a heavy metal up out of the soil—thallium. Could it be that in eating kale twice a day, embracing the purity of cleanses and vegetables, I was consuming one of the things that made it harder for my body to function? The irony amused the writer in me, alert to the ways we unknowingly embrace what we hope to avoid. Kale was a chore to eat, if I was being honest.

To THIS DAY, many in traditional medicine dismiss alternative practitioners as quacks who harm and take advantage of patients. Several leading medical reformers I follow on Twitter are reduced to almost childish fury by the very notion of alternative medicine and post sweeping dismissals of anything that smacks of quackery to them. Steven Salzberg, a professor of biomedical engineering at Johns Hopkins University, is one of the leading voices in mainstream medicine's war against alternative medicine. He argues that the NIH should stop funding studies of alternative medicine and clinics like the University of Maryland's Center for Integrative Medicine. The growing number of academic medical research centers for integrative medicine, he contends, is driven less by institutional belief that such medicine works than by a cynical hunger for grant money. "It's cleverly marketed, dangerous quackery," he told *The Atlantic* in 2011. "These clinics throw together a little homeopathy, a little meditation, a little voodoo, and then they add in a little accepted medicine and call it integrative medicine."

In his view, alternative medicine is anything but harmless. As Salzberg told David Freedman of *The Atlantic*, acupuncture needles carry "a real risk of infection" and a chiropractic adjustment could potentially "shear an artery in your neck, and you'll die." But these extreme examples of medical risks, though real, are incredibly rare. As Freedman put it, "A *British Medical Journal* study last year found that only 200 cases of likely acupuncture-related infection have been reported globally." And they pale compared to those that attend many Western medical practices (such as unnecessary cesarean sections and overprescribed opioids) undertaken by doctors with hardly a second thought. Indeed, in 2016 the *BMJ* estimated that medical errors were the third leading cause of death in the United States. Unnecessary chiropractic adjustments; unnecessary C-sections: which is worse? The answer depends on your point of view.

I don't mean to make light of the issue. A system that does not submit itself to double-blind trials is susceptible to the distorting convictions of not just quacks but people who are themselves misled and eager for answers. Even so, what often goes ignored are the philosophical reasons sick people search for care. When people get sick, they ask themselves: Are we parts or are we whole? Are we mechanisms or are we something more? And whatever we *are*, what do we want to *feel like we are* when we're ill? I found the idea of a middle way appealing. Couldn't I have the best of both worlds?

When it comes to chronic illness, both Western and alternative medicine read the body of the patient metaphorically. Western medicine is based on one kind of metaphor—the body is a car, and its parts need upkeep, piece by piece. It is not a metaphor that works well for chronically ill patients, whose parts cannot be "fixed." Alternative medicine offers a more appealing metaphor: the body is an ecosystem and caring for it as a whole—making the patient feel seen—is crucial. Alternative medicine may derive some of its power from its metaphors, but, as any poet knows, good and bad metaphors shape reality for better or for ill. In this case, when deployed well, alternative medicine may be such a good metaphor it literally changes the physiology of patients: healing as metaphor.

Traditional medical doctors point to the fact that most symptoms wax and wane, so the relief that a patient experiences following an appointment with an acupuncturist, for example, would probably have occurred even in the absence of that visit. Or might be due to the placebo effect. But evidence exists that the functional approach leads to measurable positive outcomes. In 2019, a study of patients at a clinic in Iran found that "laughter yoga"—gentle yoga that includes laughing—was more effective than anti-anxiety medication in controlling symptoms of irritable bowel syndrome, which are worsened by stress. Studies of acupuncture have shown that certain treatments can balance your autonomic nervous system, helping shut down your hyper-stimulated sympathetic nervous system—designed to help you evade predators and perform challenging mental tasks—and kick in your parasympathetic system, which helps your body restore and repair. (After my acupuncture appointments, I would go home and fall into sound sleep for hours.)

One of the integrative doctors I saw—a gentle, data-obsessed type who bicycled everywhere—told me he wanted to test me for Lyme disease. I'd never had a bull's-eye rash, I said. Not everyone gets them, he told me; have you ever been tested? I hadn't. The possibility that I had Lyme disease seemed remote. When the results came back, they were negative, but he told me he thought I should get a second, more-sensitive test. I shrugged off the idea. My other doctors, like Dr. K, were focused on the viruses that *were* showing up on my test results, which seemed a more plausible cause of my problems. I suppose in this sense they, like the conventional doctors I saw, also missed something important.

In this period of my quest, the integrative doctors I saw were more instrumental to my emotional well-being than any Western doctor I saw. But I understood that I was making a guinea pig out of myself. That is, I appreciated the fact that the integrative doctors I saw seemed to believe in the reality I described, but I also knew that their professed belief was the key to their financial success, just as fifteen-minute appointments were the model on which insurance-based conventional medicine ran.

BY THE HOLIDAY SEASON—eating fewer and fewer foods, dumping all my chemical-ridden skin-care products in the trash, gathering the plastic in our house into an enormous garbage can—I was beginning to feel like the character in Todd Haynes's film *Safe* who ends up living in a kind of sterile igloo to try to protect herself from environmental allergies. Jim listened calmly one night as I paced in the kitchen, spiraling into anxiety, and suggested I pinpoint what was known piece by piece.

Twice a day, I lined the bottles of pills and supplements along our kitchen countertop while the clock ticked loudly behind me. The supplement bottles were almost all made of plastic, with white tops that screwed off easily. *Good thing we don't have kids*, I thought. First, I took the fish oil capsules, which were huge—hard to swallow if I didn't concentrate on getting a big enough gulp of water.

Then I went through the supplements—glutathione, which reduced inflammation and helped detoxify my body (it helped me more than any other supplement I took); curcumin (concentrated turmeric), also to reduce inflammation; methylated folate and B_{12} because of the MTHFR polymorphisms; vitamin D; probiotics; pancreatic enzymes (to help absorb nutrients from my food); grapefruit seed extract; licorice to help with adrenal fatigue; and more. By the tenth pill I would start to gag. I could picture the gelatinous capsules sliding down my throat into my empty stomach, where they slowly dissolved. Was I further harming myself? I didn't have the luxury of wondering that: from my uncomfortable perch at the edge of medical understanding, I had to experiment.

As my flare subsided, I kept up with the dry brushing. The metered portions of nondairy kefir. The flaxseeds and the cinnamon. The monitoring of my lab results. Then, as I was staring at my array of pill bottles one morning, a flicker of rebellion stirred in me. I had improved on the new regimen. But had I become trapped in my identity as a sick person, someone afraid of living? If my mission in life had been reduced to being well at all costs, then the illness had won.

The next day, my friend Gina asked me how I was. We were sitting with organic pour-overs at the kind of Brooklyn place that sells Paleo-friendly almond-flour muffins. I recited the latest details (my thyroid antibodies were suddenly higher than ever, and what was with the maddening itching along my legs?) and then stopped. I sounded, I realized, like every other health-obsessed narcissist. My search for clinical illumination had grown claustrophobic. I had a diagnosis—Hashimoto's disease—but now it also seemed to have *me*. "I'm OK," I said. "I'm actually OK," hoping it was true.

You cannot muscle your way to health when you are chronically ill. Rather, one way of coming to terms with an amorphous systemic disease is recognizing that you are sick, that the illness will come and go, and that it is not the kind of illness you can conquer. Once you're feeling OK-ish, trying to be the Best Patient in the World all the time can become an isolating preoccupation. I thought about my aunts and the matter-of-fact way that they lived with their illnesses as something to deal with, but not something to fuss over. At times I might have to temper my own fanatical pursuit of wellness. On the model of D. W. Winnicott's good-enough mother, the trick was to be a good-enough patient. For me, that meant embracing the best of alternative and conventional medicine while resisting the dream of nostalgic purity that could lead me to believe I could overcome all my problems through diet and detoxification alone.

On our way to a movie that week, Jim and I saw a gluten-free pizza place. Inside, I happily inhaled the smell of cheese and baking dough. "I'll take that," I said, pointing to an oily vegetable-and-cheese gluten-free slice. "There's a vegan one—don't you want that?" Jim asked. I looked at the thin, puckering yellow counterfeit. It looked like old Silly Putty. I shook my head. "Go crazy," he said.

SEVEN

DOWNWARD SPIRAL

As winter progressed and so did my illness, Jim and I fought. What he *didn't* do, such as come to the doctors with me, took on oversized importance. What he did do (stick by me, believe me) was less obvious to me, or never enough. At times my anger about what was happening settled on him: I felt a profound sense of betrayal that he did not seem to feel the urgency of my suffering. He seemed to credit my testimony fully, even to reflect that I was quite sick, in a way that few people did. But he didn't seem to think he needed to help solve the mystery of what was afflicting me. Was it fair of me to ask this of him? Was it fair to say, *I want you to feel some of this as vividly as I do?*

On my message boards a recurrent theme was having a partner who didn't help, who didn't get it, who even judged and blamed. Even partners who did help often couldn't feel the wave of need engulfing the ill person. And my god, the need. It felt shameful to *need* other people so much. I needed practical help, often, including financial assistance paying my doctors. But I also needed—or thought I needed—recognition of what I was going through. At the best of times, it is hard to be the partner of someone ill, at once up close to the problem and permanently on the other side of the glass from it. I had the sense that Jim felt both guilt that I was sick while he was not and that he didn't want to look too closely at what I was enduring, because it spoke to his own vulnerability.

Jim was a person who thought his way through challenging situations before he felt his way through them. He was rational, evidence based, coolheaded in the face of conventional wisdom, eager to disbelieve—and argue with—received ideas, especially if they had any air of rejecting science in favor of some otherwise-known truth. He wasn't someone who would slow down, tune in, say, *Are you OK? Do you need anything?* But he had a gift for being very present. Although caretaking was not his strength, he cooked for me with real attention after a surgery when I was deeply nauseated by the prospect of most food.

One Friday, the month after I'd first seen Dr. E, I started a fight with Jim when he got home from work. I didn't feel well; he was busy getting ready for a short work trip to Seattle. I began needling him, trying to show him that he was in the wrong. All it did was make me feel worse. Your need, when you are sick, can squeeze up inside your chest, balling its way up and out of your throat. I pictured it as a thick, viscous, toxic gel that slid out of me at moments when nothing else could.

Jim flew back to New York two days after our squabble. While his plane was still in the air, I got a call from my sister-in-law. "Where's Jim?" she asked. "His dad collapsed and is in the hospital." His father had bleeding in his brain, caused, doctors initially thought, by an unstable hemorrhagic cavernoma. When Jim landed, we rushed to Connecticut. As we drove, I thought of the hours his father had spent teaching me how to drive when my own mother was ill so that I could take her to doctor appointments. (Having grown up in New York City, I was a late driver.)

The next day, Jim's father returned to consciousness. Incredibly, he recovered almost totally for a few months. The doctors said his brain was absorbing back most of the blood. Soon he was doing physical therapy and golfing. He and Jim's mom came to visit us for a few days. In his kind, generous way, he continued to ask how I was feeling and whether it was OK for me to eat this or that. I wanted to tell him not to worry about *me*. A few weeks after visiting us, he collapsed again. This time he never fully recovered. Now the doctors thought he had a brain tumor from metastatic melanoma. The prognosis was not good.

I was getting sicker even as Jim's father's outcome began to look worse, and it became hard for us to connect. I needed more than he could give. It was, I knew, simply too much for Jim, but his remoteness was devastating. While I wrestled with the dawning reality that something was very wrong with me, he was not there to assure me (even falsely) that it was going to be OK, that he was on my side, that we would figure it out. These were the things I desperately wanted to hear, true or not. But I knew I could not ask for comfort at a moment when he was strained by his father's grave illness. I understood firsthand, from my mother's cancer diagnosis, how shocking the sudden encounter with a parent's mortality is, and my heart hurt for him and his family. One day when I was reading, I came across something Tolstoy said about Ivan Ilyich: "What he longed for was impossible, but still he longed for it." Jim's father passed away a few days before Christmas. It was a mournful holiday.

In January 2013, I moved to Los Angeles for a semester. I had received a fellowship to teach a class as an honorary chair of writing at Scripps College in the town of Claremont, situated east of the city. A friend had a guesthouse in Echo Park, about forty minutes from campus, that he was willing to rent to me.

It was a piece of luck to have received this visiting position. Energized by my good fortune, I imagined myself like Keats, heading for the restorative warm winds that bring health, though I hoped—unlike Keats—for a successful rehabilitation, fueled by bee pollen supplements and green juices and spirulina, by the methylated B_{12} and folate I was now taking.

The guesthouse was airy and bright, with a small kumquat tree just outside the living room's picture window. The bedroom looked out across a lush green valley. Jim was going to stay in Brooklyn. He needed time to recover from his father's death. After our fighting, a short time apart seemed manageable, maybe even a good thing.

Meanwhile: sunshine, good weather, hiking, gluten-free cafés, time to write and read and think in a new place—a sanitarium-style winter seemed ideal for my project of self-healing. I pinched myself at my good fortune.

Those first days, the sun sparkled reassuringly. It felt good on my skin. The grocery store produce appeared to have been rendered in Technicolor. The neighborhood I lived in was full of artisanal bakeries, juice bars, palm trees, and undulating hilly walking trails. I loved being alone in my cottage, making my chia-seed smoothies and roasting sweet potatoes and writing. The solitude felt nourishing, and for once my specialized diet and my elaborate regimen of self-care—the dry-brushing and all that—seemed normal rather than odd. I met a novelist friend for dinner the night I arrived, and she took me to a nearby restaurant just off Sunset Boulevard. When I launched apologetically into my list of food allergies, the waiter brightened and said, "In fact, *all* our dishes are gluten-free!"

I had the sense of expansive waste that came with being alone in a new city, hours I could fill with reading and longing, which seemed to promise a spiritual recuperation. For a few days, I was troubled by the prospect of joy—awakened to my own mind. When, I wondered, had I last yearned for something other than simply feeling better?

One morning, a few weeks after I'd arrived, after I'd had my coffee in my tiny garden beside the kumquat tree, little electric shocks began traveling up and down my legs and arms. Zap. Then another zap. Then zap-zap. They migrated, so I never knew when or where they were coming next. My upper arm, my calf, my inner thighs. *Not again,* I thought.

The zapping shocks had recurred periodically since I'd first had them right after I graduated from college. Back then, they came on after I showered or as I walked to work, the shocks flickering up and down my legs. When I stopped to rub my calves against a parking meter, I worried that I must look as though I was performing an eccentric masturbatory act. Typically, the zapping stopped as suddenly as it had started, thirty minutes after it had begun.

For years, the zapping recurred every summer and fall. It felt like an intense form of itching, so I saw my dermatologist, who wasn't sure what the problem was beyond dry skin. Something about water set the shocks off: taking a shower or going swimming ended in agony. Instead, I washed my hair in the sink. Online, I found a few other people who had a version of them. Some had been diagnosed with a water allergy, and like me they resorted to taking sponge baths. Unlike these people, though, I was fine for months or years at a time, and water was not always a trigger. In fact, the only reliable thing about the shocks was that they started in the morning and were worse in humid weather. But I hadn't had them for a year, and I'd hoped whatever it was had gone away for good.

Now they were more intense than ever. The only thing that helped was rubbing my arms and legs very quickly, as if I were trying to warm up. If I didn't rub my skin, the sensation crescendoed into a burning pain so severe that I wished I could flay off the skin in long swaths.

That Sunday, I took a barre exercise class at a trendy place on Sunset in Silver Lake. I stood at the front of the room with several lanky bottle blondes beside me, all adorned in leggings and eighties-inspired workout tops, the décor carefully done in a hipster spa palette. An actress from the television show *The Office* stood just behind me. As we held two-pound weights and performed tiny arm lifts to carefully curated music, the shocks began—zap on the upper left arm, then zap, zap along the right calf.

I tried ignoring them. But soon I was reduced to shifting the weights into one hand and assiduously rubbing my legs and arms with the other, which for some reason made the sensation bearable. The shocks intensified. My leg twitched. Then my left arm flailed outward, convulsing as if it had received a dose of electricity.

For fuck's sake, I thought, and I ducked out of the class, flushed and embarrassed.

That spring in LA, the episodes came every morning and lasted longer than the usual thirty minutes. They now stretched to an hour, then two hours; then three hours, so that the entire morning was a torture I steeled myself to endure. I couldn't work. Instead, I squirmed on the couch, watching TV to distract myself from the worst of the pain as a firestorm passed over my body. Sometimes I read message boards where other people were complaining about the same problem. I tried different detergents and different leggings. Often, I wept in despair and pain.

One morning, after I had rubbed my legs, I noticed tiny red marks all over them. When I consulted Google, I learned that these were petechiae, or hemorrhages of tiny capillaries. Their presence could suggest an underlying medical issue. I'd never before had these marks. Now I started noticing strange bruises and petechiae all over my body—on my neck, my stomach, my legs. My fatigue was getting worse, too. One Wednesday, on my weekly drive to Scripps, I nodded off on a clean stretch of I-10, fifteen minutes into my drive, before I startled awake. Seconds later my eyes again grew heavy, the car drifting right. I found myself snapping alert, heart pounding.

That day, the shocks started while I was teaching my workshop. I gazed out at the room, trying not to flinch, then surreptitiously rubbed my legs under the table. The relief was so extreme it was almost like orgasm—a flooding sense of heat as the shocks darting over my body subsided.

"Professor?" a student was saying. The class was regarding me with curiosity and concern. "Did you hear my question?"

MY DAYS IN CALIFORNIA were repetitive. I woke up early; I went for a walk in Elysian Park, which had lovely views. On the way back to the guesthouse, I would stop at the tiny artisanal greengrocer Cookbook—which sells the most beautiful produce I've ever seen, in pristine handfuls—to buy a five-dollar grapefruit, a box of glistening, plump dates. How could I fail to get better if I spent half my paycheck on sustainably sourced organic produce? Back at the guesthouse, I made a smoothie or ate my homemade chia and flaxseed pudding and tried to write. The writing wasn't going well. The poems were dull; the essay I was working on wouldn't come.

Today, I remember very little about those months, other than what I know from the notes I took at the time. I saw almost no one; I found it exhausting to talk to new people.

One morning, I woke up early. Something was especially wrong. I made a smoothie, forcing myself to eat. I got dressed for my walk, going through the motions, my limbs like sandbags. There was a sharp pain in my abdomen. Sitting on the couch to catch my breath, I called Jim in Brooklyn.

"I don't think I'm OK," I said.

The pain got so severe I almost passed out. Instead, I threw up. When I picked up the phone again, Jim was talking but the sound of his voice hurt my head, and I asked him to sit in silence on the phone as I drove to CVS for ibuprofen. The pain made it hard to walk, but somehow, with Jim encouraging me onward, I hobbled from the parking lot to the medicine aisle, paid, and drove home again, where I called the doctor, made an appointment, took two ibuprofens, and fell asleep.

When I woke, I felt fine. I wondered briefly if it had all been a dream—an omen. I called a gynecologist for an emergency consultation. It was a sunny, clear, cool day, but I was worried about what had happened. Driving on Sunset, I approached a small intersection—I had the green light—going about thirty miles an hour, when a young man with two friends in a red Volkswagen Jetta drove through the intersection straight into me, T-boning the car. My head whipped forward and back. When my brain caught up with what had just happened, I saw that the entire front of my car was totaled. I was lucky I hadn't been two feet farther along. The rest of the day was spent exchanging insurance— the other driver was at fault, as he acknowledged—getting a tow truck, and renting a car. I was unhurt. But the next morning, the shocks and the pain were worse than ever.

When I saw the doctor two weeks later, she found nothing abnormal, but she ventured that the episode of abdominal pain was related to my history of endometriosis. She told me I should be trying harder to get pregnant; time was not on my side. It was challenging for patients with endometriosis to get pregnant, she reminded me, for reasons that likely had to do with inflammation interfering in the process of implantation.

I did not need her to tell me that time was not on my side. I was in my midthirties, and I wanted to have a child. Jim and I had started trying when we got back together in 2010. Two years later, my friends were all having children and we weren't. As I grew sicker, a quality of sad fragility had set in. Getting pregnant seemed impossible, out of grasp. But I wanted children so much that once I'd started feeling a little better, we had consulted a fertility specialist, who advised trying assisted reproductive techniques. Was this the time, though? We wanted to wait for me to be strong enough to get through the pregnancy.

When my doctor spoke, some part of me was astonished by her cruelty. But I also experienced a sting of pride that I understood the existential absurdity of her admonishment and she did not. She had not, like me, spent months waking in a body that kept confronting her with the stubbornness of its predicament. She had not, like me, crossed into the strange field that borders the road we think we walk. From the utter remove of this field one clearly sees the fictiveness of the road, with its illusion of destination. So extreme is the removal that it leads the sick person to feel that *she* is the healthy one and the healthy are the diseased, or at least the deluded.

Of course, I still had some hope about my future, about children, like the character in the novel who senses her fate yet proceeds despite it, plunging deeper into her predicament.

THE SEMESTER SLOGGED ALONG. I tried to write. I cooked vegetables and chicken and stared at the computer screen in the long balmy evenings, but the words kept slipping off the page as if through a sleeve in time.

I went gray with frustration at the remoteness of my own mind, my very selfhood. I watched TV, and I took walks, and I did physical therapy, and somehow the days passed. But I had a sense that my battery was drained. I was coming up against a physical reality that conflicted with my assumptions that I would, by now, be on an upward trajectory. ("I don't believe I will get better," Daudet wrote, ". . . yet I always behave as if my damned pains were going to disappear by tomorrow morning.")

One late afternoon, I went to see a film at the independent movie theater in Los Feliz. Sitting in the dark with three other people who for whatever reason had had to flee their lives that day, I sat and wept at the corny resolution scene. It wasn't clear to me why I was weeping—the movie was not very good. But I realized, walking home, that the problems facing the protagonists were connected to *life*, whereas my problem was the small death of each day.

I was beginning to feel a kind of panic I could neither express nor contain. I didn't know the words with which to describe it. There was something invisible about it, mute, flattening.

Not everyone feels this way about illness—or rather, not every illness leads to this feeling. "The knowledge that you're ill is one of the momentous experiences in life," Anatole Broyard wrote, speaking of being "galvanized" by his diagnosis of prostate cancer in *Intoxicated by My Illness*. Susan Sontag told *The New York Times* that her cancer diagnosis had "added a fierce intensity to my life, and that's been pleasurable." But there was nothing galvanizing or fiercely intense about my experience. It was more like a soul going limp, a steady drain of energy and of will.

People whose illness has no name get little sympathy. News of a friend or family member's fresh diagnosis often brings with it what the poet Christian Wiman calls "that little shiver of pleasure-horror" which, as he puts it, is your self realizing, "*I'm going to die!*" But when the terms of your disease are unclear even to doctors, that pain-shiver doesn't come. The people around you might feel the loosest kind of tremble within. But the tremble quickly settles into disbelief rather than the "promiscuous sympathy" Wiman experienced as a young person diagnosed with cancer.

Indeed, you may be the object of a promiscuous antipathy.

But wasn't it dire to slide slowly down into quicksand as those around you look away?

It is when we lose longing that we lose being. Depressives know this. At my most subdued, I thought of this stanza by the poet George Herbert describing his experience of a season of spiritual despair that sounds a lot like clinical depression:

> Who would have thought my shriveled heart
> Could have recovered greenness? It was gone

Quite underground; as flowers depart
To see their mother-root, when they have blown,
   Where they together
   All the hard weather,
Dead to the world, keep house unknown.

I, too, had gone underground. I was finding it more and more impossible to summon up the sparks of will that make a writer write. The hard weather had me keeping house unknown. I still had a strange sense of being an impostor. *I'm not myself,* I kept thinking. *But then who am I? And who is this "I" who knows that "I" am not "myself"?*

Although Jim stuck by me, it was hard to feel connected. In my illness I was moored in an unreachable northern realm, exiled to an invisible kingdom, and it made me angry. I wanted to rejoin the throngs.

In dark moments I continued to wonder if the wrongness *was* me. Perhaps it *was* a problem of character that made me feel this way. I didn't believe this to be true, but I had no explanations for my symptoms and little corroboration in my lab work. I still wonder if patients with a well-understood disease feel this way. Are these questions particular to—and intensified by—uncertainty, or are they a feature of any ongoing experience of ill health? Or both?

In May, Jim came to pick me up and pack my things. We were planning to take a road trip to the sites of some of the Anasazi cliff dwellings in Utah, New Mexico, and Arizona, before flying back to New York. For days we drove the empty flat roads of the West, zooming past monumental rock formations that seemed to speak a language of their own, a language of silence, persistence, and stillness that made my illness and personhood seem nothing more than a fleck in the great storm of time. I wondered whether I could—even *should*—accept the fact that my body was slowly and inexorably failing.

At one of the Anasazi sites, we climbed down to the bottom of a steep canyon to see some dwellings carved deep in the rock face. We started later than we should have, and the sun was already high and strong. It was a dry June day that was unusually hot even for the Southwest. The steep descent along a path that switchbacked down the canyon wall wasn't too hard, still shaded by the cliffs. We lingered at the base of the canyon, where trees clustered by a rivulet, taking in the otherworldliness of the place and studying the mysterious domiciles the Anasazi had built in the rock.

By the time we started back up the canyon, the sun was out in full force and the shade was gone. To get to our car, we had to climb three quarters of a mile up the cliff trail. Soon my muscles burned and my heart was racing. The heat built inside me, so that it felt like my skin was swelling. The light made my eyes hurt. I paused at every turn to rest and wipe the sweat away. An older German couple who looked to be in their late sixties passed us easily.

Two thirds of the way to the top, I ran out of water. I got woozy; the world swam. We stopped to lean against the wall under one tiny outcrop that provided shadow. The heat had become a dimension of its own. I was drowning in its obscene strength.

"I don't know if I can make it," I said to Jim, flashing on the stories I'd read of hikers who died of dehydration a half mile from the trail head.

"OK," he said. "Let's rest. You don't look great."

He gave me his water. He took my arm and slowly we made our way to the top, where my legs began shaking. When we got in the car, I shivered and shook uncontrollably. Jim offered me a bottle of water from the cooler but my hands were shaking, too, and I couldn't take the top off.

"Is this normal?" I asked.

He was shading his face, looking at our map, having had to do all the driving. He sighed. "No, I don't think so," he said quietly.

The shivering lasted until we got to the hotel room, until I sat in the pool and let my muscles go limp, collapsing in a fugue of exhaustion. I lay in bed that night feeling ashamed of my foolish wish to have a child. I could barely take care of myself.

"I want a chip implanted in my wrist," I told Jim when we got home to Brooklyn later that week, "that could give a readout of the problems in my body. I just want a device to explain what is happening on a cellular level each day. If only there were a display code—'Error 42!'—with a manual that explained what was wrong, I could bear it."

Jim laughed, because he knew my general need for control. And then he sobered and said, "I can imagine."

punitive fantasies
gendered expression

EIGHT

THE WOMAN PROBLEM

One of the punitive fantasies—to borrow Susan Sontag's phrasing—society has long held about women who are ill is that their unwellness is mainly in their heads. The stereotype of the sickly woman whose disease is strictly psychological still holds today, when examples in medical literature of "problem patients" are nearly always women. And so it is a truth universally acknowledged among the chronically ill that a young woman in possession of vague symptoms like fatigue and pain will be in search of a doctor who believes she is actually *sick*. More than 45 percent of autoimmune disease patients, a survey by the Autoimmune Association found, "have been labeled hypochondriacs in the earliest stages of their illness." Of the nearly one hundred women I interviewed, all of whom were eventually diagnosed with an autoimmune disease or another concrete illness, more than 90 percent had been encouraged to seek treatment for anxiety or depression by doctors who told them nothing physical was wrong with them.

Around the time I got sick, my grandmother and my father told me at a family gathering how much my great-aunt, who died in the early 2000s, had enjoyed being ill herself. She was a frail, thin artist with a big smile who was often in bed when I visited her. I remember liking her very much, and I remember, too, that she had a habit of talking about her symptoms, musing about what was happening in her body. In the decade since her death, several of my aunts were diagnosed with autoimmune disorders, and it seems plausible that my great-aunt had had a genuine illness. But some in our family believed that she simply craved attention.

The assumption that women are hypochondriacs is prevalent in cases of a disease of uncertain origin: the combination of modern physicians' distaste for uncertainty and society's unconscious bias against women makes it easy for health workers today to categorize vague symptoms as signs of anxiety or depression. Yet the facts themselves suggest that doctors should pay special attention to young women with symptoms that come and go. Studies tell us that women are the overwhelming sufferers of autoimmune diseases, that autoimmune diseases are increasingly common, and that they are notoriously hard to identify in blood work early on. Estimates suggest that as many as one in four women will develop an autoimmune disease; a rational doctor, presented with a patient who feels unwell and has a family history of autoimmunity, ought to think, *This might be one of those patients.* Instead, on the message boards I visited, and from the women I interviewed, I heard story after story of women being dismissed by physicians.

In the middle of the night, when I woke in the dark with my heart pounding, what *really* terrified me was the conviction that my doctors did not believe me, and so I would never have partners in my search for answers—and treatments. How could I get better if no one thought I was sick?

. . .

BEFORE I'D GOTTEN SICK, I assumed that the medical system would care for me as well as it possibly could, with the entire objective rigor science could muster. As a previously healthy upper-middle-class white cis woman—a person of privilege, in other words—I had been given, in my brief encounters with medicine, no reason to suppose otherwise. But as I became more entangled in the medical system, I discovered that I was deeply mistaken. It remains remarkably challenging for women to get consistent access to first-rate care. Medicine treats women differently from the way it treats men, as Barbara Ehrenreich and Deirdre English show in *For Her Own Good: Two Centuries of the Experts' Advice to Women*, and gender has real implications for medical care—mostly negative ones, if you're a woman.

Until recently, most medical research was performed almost exclusively on cisgender men and male animals. A 2011 study found that male mice were overwhelmingly used in four fifths of the fields studied. Researchers do not include female mice in their studies, *The New York Times* noted, because of concern that "the hormonal cycles of female animals would add variability and skew study results."

And so research has failed to consider differences in male and female biology, including disparities in how people of different sexes respond to pharmaceutical drugs—due to variations in metabolism, body fat percentages, and enzyme activity. Low-dose aspirin lowers the risk of heart attack in men, but it has no impact on heart disease risk for women under sixty-five. Beta-blockers may place women with hypertension at a greater risk of heart attack, a 2020 study found. (The authors conducted the study after realizing that women were historically underrepresented in clinical studies of beta-blockers.) Women have more complications from anesthesia. In 2001, the Institute of Medicine published a report called *Exploring the Biological Contributions to Human*

Health—Does Sex Matter? "It matters," the report concluded, "in ways that we did not expect. Undoubtedly, it also matters in ways that we have not begun to imagine." But little changed. The result is a profound lack of knowledge. As recently as 2014, Dr. Janine Austin Clayton, the associate director for women's health research at the NIH, told *The New York Times*, "We literally know less about every aspect of female biology compared to male biology."

As a consequence, some drugs that receive FDA approval are later discovered to be unusually harmful for women or to require different dosages than the one that was approved. One such drug is Ambien, which is metabolized so much more slowly by women than by men that women were getting into car accidents the morning after taking it. In 2013, the FDA required the manufacturer to reduce the approved dose for women by a remarkable 50 percent. "Of the FDA-approved drugs that had been pulled from the market between 1997 and 2001 because they were found to have 'unacceptable health risks,'" Maya Dusenbery reports in *Doing Harm: The Truth About How Bad Medicine and Lazy Science Leave Women Dismissed, Misdiagnosed, and Sick*, "eight out of ten were more dangerous to women than to men." In the current research system, little work is done to identify whether sex differences might mean that some drugs work well for men but not women, or to understand how they might work for transgender people in different phases of medical transitioning. This failure both to produce and to analyze sex- and gender-based data constitutes a remarkable oversight.

But medicine has not simply neglected to research women's health; it has also failed to treat women who are sick. One study found that women in various ERs were 13 to 25 percent less likely to receive opioid painkillers (the strongest painkiller medicine has) than men were. A study of women presenting with signs of heart attack found that they underwent cardiac catheterization—a procedure that helps identify whether heart disease is present—half as often as men. A 2014 study in Sweden found that women wait an average of fifteen minutes longer to be seen in emergency rooms than men do.

The central issue is that physicians tend not to see women's self-reports of illness symptoms as valid. When a female patient complains of pain or discomfort, her testimony is viewed as a gendered expression of a subjective emotional issue rather than a reflection of a "hard" objective physiological reality. Even when it comes to a disease as grave as cancer, a woman's testimony about what she is experiencing is seen as an exaggeration. You can guess what happens, then, when doctors cannot identify the source of the symptoms. One young woman I interviewed told me, "I wish doctors had just looked me in the eye and said, 'I don't know what's wrong with you. But I believe you. And one day we'll figure it out.' I would have had so much more confidence in that person. To have the arrogance to believe we know everything about everything! The number of physicians who said, 'There's nothing wrong with you. You're just depressed'—well, it was so demeaning."

The statistics of undertreatment and misdiagnosis are even more stark when it comes to treatment of women of color. Studies routinely show that Black and Latinx patients are undertreated for symptoms compared with white patients. Black women's complaints are dismissed, with devastating consequences. For example, Black women were even less likely than white women to be referred for cardiac catherization, another study indicated. And a 2020 report released by the Centers for Disease Control and Prevention's National Center for Health Statistics found that Black women in the United States were 2.5 times more likely to die from pregnancy or delivery complications than white women.

The British philosopher Miranda Fricker uses the term "testimonial injustice" to describe the way that prejudice against a group can unfairly undermine the credibility of an individual within it. It is a distinctive kind of epistemic injustice, she argues, because it undermines the speaker's capacity as "a giver of knowledge." I shivered in recognition when I read her words: this was precisely the sense of wrong I felt after a medical encounter. It is also what the philosopher Jill Stauffer calls "ethical loneliness" in her book of the same title, about what she calls the "injustice of not being heard." Ethical loneliness is what happens when wrongs are compounded by going cruelly unacknowledged. The term speaks to the special pain of being part of a silenced group, and the pain you feel when the possibility of communication disappears simply because of your identity. The loneliness is profound.

Diana C, who was a twenty-eight-year-old content marketer living in Queens at the time I spoke with her, experienced chronic problems that doctors couldn't pinpoint. Finally, she was diagnosed with ankylosing spondylitis as well as an arteriovenous malformation of the brain, which triggered fatigue and headaches and ultimately required multiple neurosurgeries. (She is now thirty-three and works part-time as a patient advocate.) In the years leading up to her diagnosis, she saw at least ten doctors, most of whom shrugged off her symptoms once initial tests turned up few clear answers. She told me, "I don't really understand how so many doctors could think that I was making up my symptoms—did I have nothing better to do in my life than make things up? Not that they didn't do *some* research, but they didn't look deeper into the problem!" She added, "Unfortunately, anxiety is high up on their list of considerations. They check one or two things and if they don't find anything, it's anxiety. But it would be better for a doctor to say, 'I don't know what this is,' because as the patient, you're trained to trust medical authority. If they say, 'It's anxiety,' part of you will think that it *is* anxiety." Diana found it plausible that an emotional state like anxiety could make a person feel sick. But she found it hard to believe that anxiety could be an "all-encompassing, completely debilitating, can't-get-out-of-bed-for-months" problem. She paused. "Anxiety should be the very last thing they come to, after they check out every single other thing."

. . .

THE NOTION THAT SICK WOMEN are inventing their illnesses or suffering from psychosomatic disorders has a long history. But it was brought to new prominence by the nineteenth-century embrace of hysteria as a medical diagnosis in western Europe and the United States, and the subsequent ascent of Sigmund Freud's theories of the unconscious. Today, even if doctors are not explicitly thinking about (or even buying into) Freud's theories, his ideas have provided the backdrop for much of their education. A body with symptoms that are not medically identifiable is a body communicating *psychological* issues: this idea is subconsciously present in exam rooms today, even if physicians are not actively quoting Freud to their patients. Indeed, it is an idea that all of us have absorbed.

How did this come to be? The ancient Egyptians and Greeks—as my father, an Egyptologist and classicist, taught me—laid the blame for various medical conditions on women's wombs ("hystera," in Greek). Hippocratic medicine believed the the womb could "wander" and cause disease, including a condition known as "hysterical suffocation." Related concepts about diseases suffered by women made their way to late-medieval Europe. By the thirteenth century, some religious scholars saw symptoms that would later be labeled "hysteria" as a specifically female ailment caused by the devil. As one scholar puts it, "if a physician cannot identify the cause of a disease, it means that it is procured by the Devil."

In the late nineteenth century, hysteria came into wide use as a medical diagnosis. Physicians of the time initially believed that hysteria was an organic (or physical) illness, with symptoms ranging from fatigue to anxiety to abdominal pain, that was caused by the overloading of the nervous system. Many Victorian physicians believed that the womb and the recently discovered nervous system were intimately connected, making women both "product and prisoner of her reproductive system," as the scholars Charles E. Rosenberg and Carroll Smith-Rosenberg put it. (In 1870, a physician wrote that it was "as if the Almighty, in creating the female sex, had taken the uterus and built up a woman around it.") It was thought that "brain work" could literally drain energy from the uterus, making women weak and fatigued. And so many doctors drew a connection between the "epidemic" of hysteria and the rise of suffragism and women's intellectual exertions. (Among the women to receive a diagnosis of hysteria were the writers Charlotte Perkins Gilman and Alice James.) Doctors such as Silas Weir Mitchell, who pioneered the still-infamous rest cure (with which Gilman was treated), tried to treat hysteria with elaborate dietary restrictions and prescribed quiet; but their patients didn't get better.

Frustrated by their recalcitrant female patients, male physicians came to see hysteria as a manifestation of underlying emotional issues—the now-familiar idea that a body speaks hidden emotional truths through physical symptoms.

The man who brought this idea into the mainstream, of course, was Sigmund Freud. Like other doctors, including his teacher Jean-Martin Charcot, a French neurologist, he originally believed that his hysterical patients were suffering from a physical disease. But when they failed to get better under his care, he came to believe that their symptoms were an expression of trauma such as sexual assault, or repressed libidinal urges, as the medical historian Anne Harrington recounts in *The Cure Within*. For Freud, the body was speaking a truth, but it was a truth about the patient's unconscious. And only the doctor could interpret what that truth was; as Harrington writes, "From now on, the doctor's interpretations of the coded messages from the body . . . would emphatically trump that of the patient, and it would do so even if (sometimes especially if) the patient resisted or denied those interpretations." Psychoanalysis was the creative process by which an analyst uncovered what the mind knew but couldn't admit.

And there you have it: a framework in which the doctor became the expert on the woman's symptoms, and the more a woman insisted on their reality, the more likely it was those symptoms were evidence of repressed psychic conflicts, of something obdurate and maladjusted in her psyche. As Harrington notes, after Freud, a patient was no longer "the best judge of what was going on with her body" and "should not necessarily be allowed the last word."

Though Freud's views on hysteria are no longer in the ascendant, his intellectual framework influences us to this day. If a female patient fails to get better, the problem lies with *her*, we continue to think (subconsciously). Indeed, the notion that the female body is often expressing psychological distress still powerfully animates medical thinking, though it has been relabeled several times—first as "Briquet's syndrome" and then, in the 1920s, as what the Viennese psychoanalyst Wilhelm Stekel called "somatization" (a "process by which neurotic conflicts appear as a physical disorder)," and most recently, as what the *Diagnostic and Statistical Manual of Mental Disorders* (*DSM*) calls "somatoform disorders," which are often wastepaper-basket diagnoses doctors use when they can't figure out what's wrong with a female patient. These disorders are so associated with gender, as Dusenbery points out, that medical students sometimes memorize them using the acronym "SDBLVP": "Somatization Disorder Besets Ladies and Vexes Physicians."

As I was writing this book, a male artist I did not know, who had read some of my essays about illness, sent me multiple unsolicited emails trying to persuade me that what ailed me was in fact the consequence of suppressed emotions I had not yet been bold enough to acknowledge—an idea he had taken from John Sarno but had distorted into a worldview that failed to accommodate the possibility that I had anything medically wrong with me. When I politely resisted the notion that the answer was so simple, he doubled down, trying to portray my resistance as proof that he was correct.

IRONICALLY, A HANDFUL OF feminist thinkers helped solidify medicine's belief that hard-to-identify female illnesses are often psychological in origin by rereading the history of female illness in the nineteenth century as a history of women's psychological distress at their restricted roles. In this reading, an oppressive patriarchy, not sublimated sexual desire, was making women sick. The scholars' work articulates something deeply important about the trauma of domestic and social powerlessness. But in focusing on the psychosocial origins of hysteria, their rereading also reinforces the idea that these women did not have a biological illness. Even for many of these second-wave white feminists, women's bodies remained primarily sites of emotional and social trauma, not bodies that may have been sick with organic diseases that were medically misunderstood (or both).

This reframing further undermined belief in women's testimony about their bodies. And so today, when a woman enters a doctor's office, with its sleek antiseptic surfaces and its precise tools, she is still entering a space that views the female body experiencing intermittent symptoms like fatigue and anxiety and pain as one that is expressing something psychological. A consequence is that poorly understood diseases are routinely psychologized by doctors, patients, and laypeople. Autoimmunity, fibromyalgia, chronic Lyme, ME/CFS—these are today's hysteria.

"Boyfriend problems?" a doctor in Los Angeles said to a friend of mine, a distinguished visual artist who has shown her work in top museums. She had entered his office complaining of ongoing pain following a freeway accident. The accident had triggered a complicated disorder of the nervous system. But the doctors she saw assumed that her pain was psychological, because she had no visible injuries. She was not diagnosed or treated for months, during which she was forced to stop painting. She began making very small drawings, using the movements that her body allowed her. It took more than a year to find a doctor who would diagnose her with, and treat her for, a pain syndrome triggered by nerve injury. Today, she is almost entirely healed and able to make art of any size she wants. One of the last times I saw her, she gave a talk about a new project in which she was making expansive and immersive print projects that took over entire architectures of decrepit and abandoned buildings, as if to demonstrate the joy of healthy embodiment.

NINE

THE IMMUNE SYSTEM
GONE AWRY

B ecause I had spent so much time searching for a matter-of-fact
cause of my suffering, I felt the need, once I got the autoimmune
thyroiditis diagnosis, to resist thinking metaphorically about what was
wrong with me. But it was impossible to get a handle on what the immune system does in our bodies without thinking symbolically.

The term "immune system" is itself a metaphor for how our immune
cells work. Our modern understanding of it as a layered network of acquired and innate immune response, in which your immune system is
in a sense tutored by its exposure to pathogens over time, was popularized in the mid-1960s, when network and systems thinking was in
the ascendancy. In 1960, the Australian virologist Frank Macfarlane
Burnet and the British biologist Peter Medawar received the Nobel
Prize for their discovery of "acquired immunological tolerance." Burnet
and Medawar showed that Paul Ehrlich's notion of the body's "horror
autotoxicus"—its aversion to self-damage—was not fixed. Rather, it

was "a matter of education," and in the education of the immune system matters could, in fact, go seriously awry.

After I started reading about autoimmune processes, I realized that my understanding of the workings of the immune system was inadequate: I hadn't studied biology since high school. I had ordered some immunology textbooks, but to make sure I was not going astray, I asked an undergraduate student at Harvard, Caleb, a biology major with a special interest in the immune system, and a friend who is a professor of biochemistry to explain the immune system to me in terms I could understand.

As I learned from them in my study sessions, the branches of the immune system are in some ways quite distinct. The innate system we are born with is our first line of defense, responding immediately to pathogens and foreign matter, deploying natural killer cells and phagocytes like macrophages and neutrophils—types of white blood cells—to fight off pathogens, frequently by ingesting or engulfing them. Acquired (also known as "adaptive") immunity is our second and more sophisticated line of defense: it mounts a response specific to the pathogen encountered, and then *remembers* those pathogens. Adaptive immune cells include B cells and T cells, which help fight off infections in concert with our innate immune system.

The primary organs of the immune system, I learned, are the bone marrow and the thymus, a soft, pinkish-gray triangular gland above our heart. (It resembles a thyme leaf, hence its name.) It is one of the few organs that grows smaller after puberty, the point at which many of our immune cells have been made. In the bone marrow and the thymus, hordes of B and T cells, named for the parts of the body from which they come, are born and educated. Both kinds of cells attack infections, heal wounds, and more. B cells make antibodies: Y-shaped proteins that target specific pathogens by locking into them in ways that bring the video game Tetris to mind. Each antibody is specific to a given pathogen;

measuring them gives doctors a record of the body's encounters—the body's memory of the foes it has faced.

With my instructors' tutelage, I came to see the immune system as a kind of college where so-called naïve immune cells grow up and—as if choosing a major—are trained to focus on a specific foreign substance. When our adaptive immune cells meet their first antigen, or bit of foreign matter, they go through structural and chemical changes. Imprinted by that antigen—as if via a kiss, Caleb said, drawing a picture of an antigen and antibody interlocked—the naïve immune cell becomes an enemy specific to it. (This is the premise behind most vaccines: they contain an altered version of a virus, to make the body produce antibodies designed specifically to lock into it.) T cells known as "T-helper cells" (technically, CD4+ T-helper lymphocytes) help ramp up the immune response in the body, stimulating B cells to produce antibodies and stimulating T killer cells, which can kill cells infected by virus.

Autoimmunity and allergies occur when immune cells mistakenly identify as pathogens things that are not threats (the thyroid, the liver, pollen, cat dander) and an immune response ensues, possibly because of what is known as "molecular mimicry." Your immune system, in trying to attack a pathogenic Epstein-Barr virus protein, ends up attacking similar-looking molecules in the body.

Immunology uses the term "regulation" to describe the body's mechanisms for calling its army of immune cells back and turning off their destructive power. As Caleb put it one day, in a metaphor I would find repeated elsewhere, "The T cells are like cadets, sent out to attack viruses. But they have little self-control, and so they are monitored by sergeants, known as 'regulatory T (T_{reg}) cells,' who tell them the attack is over and it's time to head back to the base. When the regulatory T cells aren't working, you get an out-of-control immune response, making you sicker than you need to be."

One reason people feel sick when they have an infection is that the inflammatory response of the immune system itself makes them feel sick—something I had failed to understand previously. (This is also why many people feel briefly sick after getting, for example, a COVID-19 vaccine—a vaccine, after all, is designed to provoke an immune response.) The cell that has found a virus or bacterium uses chemicals called "chemokines" and "cytokines" to recruit an inflammatory response, calling for white blood cells. These chemicals work on a gradient—like a radar signal that gets stronger and louder as you approach the targeted object. Or, as Caleb memorably described this process to me, "They're drawn to the center of the infection or wound, as if by Gandalf striking his staff and saying, 'I call you to come fight evil,'" he explained, using an analogy any *Lord of the Rings* fan could follow. The result is inflammation: blood rushes to the area and so do white blood cells and other immune cells.

The word "inflammation" comes from the Latin verb "inflammare," or "to set on fire," and it evokes the heat and redness that come with the rush of cells to a wounded or attacked area. The process is beneficial when the body deploys it appropriately, as in response to an injury. But in the long term, inflammation is harmful to tissue and cells; it can make you feel fatigued and sluggish.

Listening to Caleb, I finally had a clue to why my mornings were so awful. My immune system was acting as if I had an ongoing infection. Inside my body, inflammation reigned, worsening at night, when the immune system's production of pro-inflammatory cytokines and other T cells peaks. I woke up feeling foggy and sick. The mechanisms of the immune system, I marveled, were impossibly complex, even elegant, and still not fully knowable. A thought flickered through me: I wished I had understood more about immunity earlier in my life. I wished I had *respected* my immune system more. Had I respected it more, would I not be well today—would it not have protected me?

. . .

THE MORE I LEARNED ABOUT the immune system and autoimmune diseases, the more questions I had. The science seemed to be a road map that led every which way. I began to wonder whether I had a specific, nameable disease or a stupefying range of inflammatory responses. I also felt fresh sympathy for my doctors' frustration with patients who read up on their diseases and then announce they have answers. Overwhelmed by my research, I felt I would never find my way through the maze back to a functioning body. Theories abounded about pathways to immune dysfunction and autoimmunity—some researchers suggested that a percentage of autoimmune diseases were triggered by a virus's effects on genes; others by a degraded microbiome; others by accumulated hits to the system by pathogens; and still others by exposure to unidentified chemicals with autogenic effects. Some argued that low vitamin D or the consumption of too much salt played key roles. I had recently had blood work done that showed many anomalies in my immune response. But why? Was the root cause an immune system gone amok, stressed by toxic modernity and a flawed microbiome? What role was played by the three viruses—Epstein-Barr virus, CMV, and parvovirus—I had had at once? Could the cause be an as-yet-unknown infection my immune system could not clear? How would I ever tease the causes of my symptoms apart?

Of course, many immune-mediated diseases have a genetic component. As Moises Velasquez-Manoff points out in *An Epidemic of Absence: A New Way of Understanding Allergies and Autoimmune Diseases,* all that is necessary to "produce these disorders . . . is the removal of a single critical component of the immune system." In 1982, he reports, an infant died of a multi-organ disease in Portland, Oregon, after seventeen other male babies in his family had died, too. Researchers realized that these children had an autoimmune disease caused by a mutation on the

X chromosome involving a gene named "FOXP3." The gene helps with the production and function of the regulatory T cells, or sergeant cells, that tell other immune cells to stop fighting infection. Its malfunction can result in an ongoing state of inflammation. (This particular disease is more common in men than in women, because people who are assigned male at birth have only one X chromosome; the mutation will not be balanced out by a nonmutated second X chromosome.) By playing around with genes that affect our T_{reg} cells, researchers were able to produce autoimmune disorders in further studies.

Today, nearly one hundred genetic variations associated with lupus have been identified. Nir Hacohen, an immunologist and geneticist at the Broad Institute in Cambridge, Massachusetts, once showed me a bright screen full of colorful data mapping the mutations on the genome that are associated with the disorder. There were more than I could quickly count.

At the same time, studies of twins tell us that genetics are not the whole story; at most they're a contributing factor to autoimmune disease. The other major factor is environment. Since the 1950s, the prevalence of autoimmune diseases has risen in developed Western countries while rates of infectious disease (before COVID, at least) have been declining, thanks to vaccines, antibiotics, improved hygiene, and increased wealth. Rates of autoimmune diseases are not as high in less developed countries. For example, a 2002 study found that the rate of autoimmune type 1 diabetes in first-generation Pakistani children in the United Kingdom is approximately ten times higher than the incidence of type 1 diabetes in Pakistan.

These and other "womb-to-tomb" studies, as Noel Rose, the former director of the Johns Hopkins University Autoimmune Disease Research Center, told me, indicate that something in the Western environment (defined broadly) is causing a major shift in how our immune system functions. But why? Currently, there are many hypotheses. Some researchers ascribed the rise to our newly hygienic world: with too little to do, our immune system turns on itself. In 1989, the "hygiene hypothesis" was developed by the immunologist David Strachan, who suggested that living in small families with rising standards of cleanliness, and less exposure to infections, led to higher rates of asthma and allergy in children. We need exposure to germs, he theorized. In this line of thinking, researchers propose, the human immune system is primed to engage actively with bacteria and viruses. In the absence of major infections, the theory holds, immune cells go after harmless things instead, attacking the very body they are meant to tolerate, an idea that is laid out powerfully in Velasquez-Manoff's *An Epidemic of Absence*. The hygiene hypothesis has a moral attractive to anyone who has read myths: in trying to protect ourselves from disease, we invited it into our world.

The question, of course, is whether the relationship between the decline of infectious diseases and the rise of autoimmune diseases is one of mere correlation or actual causation. Many researchers I spoke to put little stock in the hygiene hypothesis as it was formulated, noting that there may be as many bacteria in the New York City subway system as on a farm and pointing to evidence that infections are actually key contributors to autoimmune disease. Amy Proal, a microbiologist and a founder of the PolyBio Research Foundation, told me that she believes the real question is not which germs we have, but *what activity* those germs are engaged in, and how various changing aspects of our lives may be shaping that activity.

One thing we do know is that the twentieth century led to changes in our microbiome. For decades, Westerners have used antibiotics to treat diseases they don't cure, such as colds, even though the drugs can indiscriminately kill bacteria in your gut, getting rid of "good" bacteria along with the targeted bad one. The standard American diet has also changed radically in a short period of time, becoming heavily processed. Mounting evidence suggests that processed foods disrupt our gut flora and cause increased intestinal permeability, which allows food molecules to get into the bloodstream—the so-called leaky gut—where the immune system may mount responses to them, triggering food sensitivities and autoimmune responses.

Our current diet, the microbiologists Justin and Erica Sonnenburg at Stanford University emphasize, is low in the plant fiber that feeds good bacteria, and Americans' habit of washing vegetables means we lose some of the soil-based bacteria we should be eating. As a result, our lower intestines' flora are underfed. Over time, this leads to the extinction of whole species of microbiota, an extinction that cannot be fully remedied by returning to a plant-based diet.

Add to this the fact that more C-sections are being performed in Western countries; babies born surgically miss being bathed with crucial microbes in the vaginal canal. A 2015 study from *Pediatrics* concluded that babies born by cesarean section had a "significantly increased risk of asthma, systemic connective tissue disorders, juvenile arthritis, inflammatory bowel disease, immune deficiencies, and leukemia." Suddenly the fact that I was a C-section baby seemed like a relevant piece of my history, along with the fact that I took multiple courses of antibiotics in my adolescence and twenties for colds that likely didn't need them.

At the same time, Westerners' immune systems are being exposed to a vast array of potentially hazardous chemicals in our environment, the amount of which has risen precipitously since 1950. In a single day our immune systems may confront scores of chemicals in face cream, diesel exhaust, pesticide spray, forest fires, paper, and plastics. In a 2005 study, researchers detected the presence of 287 industrial chemicals, including flame retardants, pesticides, and dioxins, in the fetal-cord blood of ten newborns. A 2021 study identified 55 chemicals never before found in humans in maternal and fetal serum samples from pregnant women. Poignantly, breast milk has been shown to contain dry-cleaning chemicals, paint thinners, and flame retardants, among other chemicals. In *The Autoimmune Epidemic*, the medical journalist Donna Jackson Nakazawa makes the case that some of these chemicals may have what she calls an "autogenic" effect on our bodies, triggering self-attack the way carcinogens trigger cancer. Indeed, Kathleen Gilbert and Neil Pumford at the Arkansas Children's Hospital have shown that trichloroethylene (TCE), a chemical used in paint and stain remover, now found in groundwater and soil, causes an autoimmune response in the T cells of genetically susceptible mice.

But we know remarkably little about whether and how chemicals may trigger immune-mediated diseases. It can be hard for researchers to get funding for studies (no potentially lucrative drugs are involved). Less than 6 percent of the NIH budget is devoted to exploring environmental effects of chemicals on humans. Chemical regulation in the United States is abysmal: the Toxic Substances Control Act of 1976, which introduced legislation aimed at regulating the use of toxic chemicals, grandfathered in 62,000 chemicals without testing them and set the bar very low for future regulation. Chemical companies in the United States are not compelled to disclose whether the substances they work with cause immunological dysfunction. A 2016 amendment to the law means that the EPA now is required to determine whether a new chemical poses a risk to humans or the environment. But the United States continues to use chemicals and pesticides banned by Europe as known carcinogens and pollutants.

WHATEVER THE ULTIMATE CAUSE (or causes) of the rise of immune-mediated diseases, it has become even clearer that infections can be significant triggers. As Noel Rose, the father of autoimmune disease research, described it to me, "genetics are the gun; a virus pulls the trigger." Researchers are beginning to identify the biomechanisms of the trigger. One day I spoke by phone with John Harley, the former director of the Center for Autoimmune Genomics and Etiology at the Cincinnati Children's Hospital Medical Center, who, along with his team, had announced a discovery: a potential piece of the genetic mechanism for how the Epstein-Barr virus triggers lupus, multiple sclerosis, and many other autoimmune diseases.

Before I got sick, I had not really understood that some viruses never go away—that, rather, they enter a latent period during which they live in our body for years, reactivating when the immune system is unable to contain them, perhaps because it is busy fighting other infections or because of the decline in immune cell production associated with aging. (Shingles, a painful rash, is caused by the reactivation of the chicken pox virus as your immune system weakens with age.) As Harley put it to me, in its latent stage the Epstein-Barr virus "hangs out in the B cells, trying to hide from the immune system, expressing itself very little"— meaning that it becomes genetically less active—only to later reactivate, sometimes causing a new bout of symptoms. Typically, this happens in people with weakened immune systems. For some reason, it was happening to me, according to my lab work. I was beginning to understand the significance of the viruses in my system that kept coming and going; I was probably not contracting them over and over, but my immune system was failing to keep them in check. The question was why? And—if these viruses *were* playing a key role in my illness—were they triggering an autoimmune reaction in me?

How and why certain viruses trigger autoimmunity in some people and not others is still not clear. "Right now, we can't tell the difference between components of the immune system that are really important in making autoimmunity and aspects that aren't," Harley told me about the state of research, likening it to the crude-tuning rather than fine-tuning knob on an old radio. But in his view, progress toward a more comprehensive understanding is under way.

What we do know is that it isn't just genes: not everyone with the genetic risk develops autoimmunity. Something has to trigger the pathological process.

Amy Proal, the microbiologist who helped found the PolyBio Research Foundation in Boston, began researching infection-initiated ill-nesses such as PTLDS and long COVID because she herself developed ME/CFS when she was a pre-med undergraduate at Georgetown University. At her sickest, she was bedridden for eight months and was told to seek psychiatric help. Eventually she recovered enough to graduate and then get a PhD in microbiology from Murdoch University in Australia. Today, she is interested, as she told me, in how pathogens dysregulate gene expression and immunity, and how the microbiome may influence chronic inflammatory diseases.

Proal believes that powerful pathogens and "successive infections" contribute to hard-to-diagnose and hard-to-treat diseases such as ME/CFS, post-treatment Lyme disease syndrome (or chronic Lyme), and long COVID. After all, she explained, "Every major pathogen down-regulates"—or in some sense inhibits—"the immune system in order to survive." So if you contract Lyme disease that goes untreated, you are susceptible to the next infection, which can "compromise the immune response further, and get into parts of your body that it might not have before," she observed. "It is almost like a snowball rolling downhill."

What complicates this even more is that we are just beginning to understand that the body is teeming with organisms, not just in our gut but in our tissues. "We are always only partly human," Proal said. Those organisms release chemical by-products that can affect many aspects of what we take to be our "self," from mood to physical well-being. Proal suspects that some inflammatory diseases are triggered by imbalances in those organisms and how those imbalances affect the immune system, as well as by pathogens that penetrate tissue and are unlikely to be found in the blood.

Unlike other researchers I met with, Proal prefers not to talk about "good" and "bad" bacteria; bacteria are organisms that can act in different ways, she pointed out to me. She is more interested in our homeostasis as a "superorganism," or "holobiont," and how and why bacteria change gene expression and become pathological, impacting our health. One general answer has to do with the dance between our immune system and our biome.

As she put it, the microbiome (whether in our gut or in other organs and tissues or, indeed, in our mouth) and our immune system are like a kindergarten class and a teacher. The class is orderly when the teacher—the immune system—is present. But if the teacher leaves the room (in this case, to fend off a virus), the normally well-behaved pupils get unruly, and the biome may misbehave. Now everyone is drawn into the bad activity, releasing chemical signals that almost appear to egg others on. As she noted, "*P. gingivalis* is the biggest cavity-driving pathogen. A lot of people have it in their mouth, and they are fine. But if your immune system isn't great, and fails to monitor it, *P. gingivalis* starts to produce biofilm-signaling molecules, and neighboring organisms are like, wait, we can join a biofilm?" (Biofilms are slimy structures inside of which bacteria live in an organized community and communicate with one another; the spongy molecular matrix that contains them helps protect them from the immune system's attacks.) And soon you've got a mouth full of cavities.

But the question remains: why do women make up approximately 80 percent of people with autoimmune diseases? An answer may lie in the replicated X chromosome (which allows for a genetic mutation to happen twice) or in the role estrogen plays in regulating the immune system. Women generally have a stronger immune response to infections and vaccines than men do. (Consider the fact that men are more likely to die from COVID than women.) Studies suggest that estrogen interacts with the adaptive immune system's B and T cells in ways that predispose it to become more "autoreactive." One review of the literature on autoimmunity noted that "many autoimmune disorders tend to affect women during periods of extensive stress, such as pregnancy, or during a great hormonal change." Studies have identified links between endocrine transition states in women and the development of lupus, multiple sclerosis, rheumatoid arthritis, and type 1 diabetes, among others;

the reproductive years, medical school teaches, put women at risk for autoimmune disease, perhaps due to the hormonal changes during and after pregnancy. During the decade surrounding menopause, studies show that women are at higher risk for developing some kinds of auto-immune diseases. Levels of anti-inflammatory cytokines decrease, and pro-inflammatory cytokines increase.

The emerging field of epigenetics has suggested that changes to gene expression during one's lifetime can also contribute to autoimmune disease. To those of us who were taught that Darwin, not Lamarck, got evolution right, the idea that the events of one's life can shape the genetics of one's child runs counter to all that we memorized for tests in high school biology. Epigenetics, though, does not refer to changes in the DNA code but to changes that can turn a gene "on" or "off." And these changes, it turns out, *can* be passed from generation to generation. Epigenetics helps determine outcomes through biological processes that impact the way proteins access or "read" a gene. Smoking, working night shifts, infections, stress, famine—all have been shown to cause epigenetic changes in the body, some of which can be passed on.

The science got complex very fast, but the image in my head, when a researcher friend taught me about epigenetics one chilly afternoon, was of a vast library containing every book in the world on a series of spinning stacks, coiled in a manner like that of DNA's double helix. (DNA has, in a sense, more information than our bodies will ever use at any given moment.) To the browser wandering by, some of those books would be more accessible than others, their spines facing out. They would be read and used more frequently, unless there was a mechanism to spin and rotate the stacks so that *other* volumes were facing the browser. In your body, one such mechanism is "methylation," which allows some parts of our genetic material to play a larger role in our lives than others. Alterations in our methylation processes may contribute to autoimmune diseases and immune function and dysfunction, although researchers are still pinpointing why and how.

But epigenetics is just one of several pathways for how biography shapes biology. Others include trauma and stress. At one point when I was sick, someone (a man) said to me, "It's always women with childhood traumas or type-A hyperstressed women who get sick. Why is that?" I didn't have an answer, but he wasn't entirely wrong. While researchers take pains to distinguish between stress (which the medical system tends to treat as observable and external) and trauma (which the medical system typically treats as an experience in the realm of psychology), both affect the immune system in complex ways that are just beginning to be understood, impacting the relationship between the sympathetic and parasympathetic nervous systems and affecting our hormones. If you imagine the hormones of the human body as a large feedback loop connecting various systems and organs—in precisely the holistic way that the Western medical system is not designed to treat—then you can begin to see how trauma and stress, by driving the body into a frequent cycle of alert, can kickstart a chain of processes that may manifest as "autonomic dysregulation," or dysregulation of our unconscious nervous system, in which small deviations in a complex chain of events lead to symptoms for the patient that are often seen as purely psychosomatic. But all too often stress or trauma is invoked as a reason not to look more closely at the biomechanisms of an illness. These invocations by healthy people imply a kind of solution to the terrifying reality of complex chronic illness: the individual is ultimately responsible for their illness, not the polity.

WHEN WE PUT ALL THIS research together, we find ourselves with multiple explanations for why autoimmune diseases, allergies, asthma, and food intolerances are rising in the West in comparison to traditional cultures. I found myself thinking of the pressure of modern life in late capitalism, with its pollution, its insecurities, its degraded food system, its overreliance on antibiotics, its endless stressors, and its weak safety nets (in the United States, at least). In each generation we compromise our microbiomes and environment and hand them off to our children, whose microbiomes and environment became further compromised by diet and chemicals.

But which causes whose illness, in what combination? Why does the patient one day feel fine and the next find pain roiling across and within her body, like an unruly spirit that needs exorcism? We do not yet know. Michael D. Lockshin, director of the Barbara Volcker Center for Women and Rheumatic Diseases at the Hospital for Special Surgery in New York City, writes in his book *The Prince at the Ruined Tower: Time, Uncertainty, and Chronic Illness*, "I now accept that uncertainty occupies a substantial part of the world in which my patients, my students, and I live. We do not need to hide it from view. It is not cause for fright. Uncertainty is just another tool that we can learn to use." Making room for uncertainty, in Lockshin's view, is a key part of the doctor's treatment of autoimmune disease.

My life as a patient changed the day I reread a letter by the nineteenth-century poet John Keats in which he offers a theory of what makes an artist great. At the time of its writing, Keats had witnessed his mother die from tuberculosis, then a poorly understood disease with an unclear cause. Soon his brother Tom and later he himself would die of the infection. In the letter, Keats—in his early twenties—tried to explain to his brothers the special quality that differentiated a great artist from a merely good one. "Negative Capability," as he termed it, is the quality "of being in uncertainties, Mysteries, doubts, without any irritable reaching after fact & reason."

I couldn't escape the sense that Keats's words about the necessity of "being in uncertainties" derived from his own experience of living with consumption's impact on his family. In fact, his formulation of negative capability seemed to be a key to living well in the face of pain. It was a profound insight of the sort that comes from witnessing loss and suffering up close. (As the chronically ill know, to be alive *is* to be in uncertainty.) I was grateful for his words, because they reminded me that I wasn't living off the known map of human experience. Rather, I had felt invisible in my illness, I realized, because American culture—and American medicine within it—largely strives to downplay the fact that we still know so little about illness. A doctor friend told me that in med school he was explicitly taught never to say "I don't know" to a patient. Uncertainty was thought to open the door to lawsuits. In the place of uncertainty, Americans have catchphrases: *Just do it. What doesn't kill you makes you stronger.* No wonder that as a patient I was bent on an "irritable reaching after fact & reason." The shadowland I lived in, forced against my will into what Keats called the great "Penetralium of mystery," was an uncomfortable and unsatisfying place, especially since I lived in a culture that promotes the importance of triumph over adversity—a culture that insists on recovery.

Writing this years later, I still feel the waves of grief that rose over me when I accepted that I had a chronic illness—that my life was permanently changed. The hardest part of what I was living through was accepting the uncertainty of whether I would ever know what was wrong with me. Someday, doctors would have a name for my illness. But in the meantime, I might become one of those people lost on the way to answers, treatments, cures—lost in the knowledge gap. There is one certainty for those of us at the edge of medical knowledge, though: we live in the gap together. As Keats witnessed more and more suffering—his brother Tom's death and the infectious illnesses sweeping London—he connected his aesthetic vision to lived experience. The world, he wrote in a letter, is "the vale of Soul-making": "Do you not see how necessary a World of Pains and troubles is to school an Intelligence and make it a soul?" Certainly, none of us would choose to suffer. But when we do suffer, we can hope that others acknowledge with us that we live without all the answers.

When I first met with my current rheumatologist (a mentee of Lockshin's), she talked about the uncertainties posed by my lab work, which was marked by abnormal results that failed to aggregate into a single specific disease entity other than autoimmune thyroiditis. She suggested I had some kind of immune dysfunction that rheumatologists hadn't yet mapped—an unspecified connective tissue disorder, perhaps. (I still had a positive ANA test.) I realized I had found the doctor I would stay with. The uncertainties did not lead her to believe I was not ill; they led her to believe science did not yet fully understand the contours of what was making me ill.

Part Two

MYSTERIES

TEN

AUTOIMMUNITY

AS METAPHOR

"I can't explain *myself*, I'm afraid, sir," said Alice, "because I'm not myself, you see."

—Lewis Carroll, *Alice's Adventures in Wonderland*

I can remember with a vividness that makes me shiver how unclear
the illness was to me, how difficult it was to get hold of its contours,
and the way the world seemed a kind of mist-filled plateau after I had
returned from California.

When I went to college, it was fashionable in literary circles to say
that the self is a construction, not a coherent experience of unity or
continuity. As a healthy person in a wood-paneled seminar room, I had
been fond of saying, rather jauntily, "Our moods do not believe in each
other," as Emerson had put it, or "Je est un autre," as Rimbaud had. But
in my new condition, I thought how wrong I had been. I now knew,
without a doubt, that there was such a thing as selfhood, because I had

lost it. It existed only in the form of dim memory, an intuition that I used to be different.

In this sense, my illness was forcing me to reckon with my identity—it had become what the scholar Miriam Bailin, in her book on Victorian sickroom scenes, calls "a forcing ground of the self." As Bailin demonstrates, fever was seen in the nineteenth century as a condition that meant something about the patient's life. In novels, a fever scene often symbolized a protagonist's spiritual crisis, a "conventional rite of passage issuing in personal, moral, or social recuperation."

For me, recuperation seemed like a fantasy. But the idea that my illness had triggered a reckoning with my self was inescapable, and I was hardly alone in my speculations. Online, in the groups I participated in on Yahoo or Facebook, I found that autoimmune diseases often led patients to confront the consequences of their own personal choices. These people identified their illness as a metaphor for their inner struggles, a verdict of some kind, even when they knew there were genetic causes. As one young woman, who had been anorexic in her teenage years, explained to me, "I almost feel like there is some sort of metaphor there with autoimmune—OK, now my body is *literally* destroying itself. With other diseases it's this kind of external thing you're fighting against. If you have cancer, you can fight your cancer. But if you have an autoimmune disease, what are you fighting against? Do you fight against your own immune system? Are 'you' your immune system? Are you the organ under attack? Who *are* you?" In her understanding of her illness, the autoimmune disease grew almost inexorably out of her former fight with her body, her conflicted embodiment.

Many patients I communicated with seemed to suspect that autoimmunity demanded that you take a closer look at who you really were. An autoimmune disease, various women in my online support groups counseled, compelled you to face the ways you were living an inauthentic life. I encountered exhausted mothers and wives who felt they did everything for those around them and nothing for themselves; women who were trapped in abusive situations; men who, longing for premodern days, had grown suspicious of microwaves or desk jobs. Poor personal choices, they all believed, had led them to this forcing ground of autoimmunity, a period of reconsidering who they are and what they have become. In the popular narratives of the late twentieth and early twenty-first centuries, then, to become autoimmune is to be seen as being personally divided, and having to heal not just your body but your mind. In *Intolerant Bodies,* Anderson and Mackay call autoimmunity "the signal pathology of the late twentieth century" for the ways it triggers a crisis of identity.

"What is the message?" I had asked myself when I saw the rash on my arm at the beach in Vietnam. It may seem like an odd question to ask about a disease. But we turn poorly understood illnesses into symbols of other things. Autoimmunity invites patients to psychologize their own symptoms like almost no other contemporary pathology does, because the fact of the immune system attacking the very body it is designed to protect seems itself metaphorical.

"All autoimmune diseases invoke the metaphor of suicide. The body destroys itself from the inside," the poet and essayist Sarah Manguso writes in her perceptive memoir *The Two Kinds of Decay.*

This sort of thinking was everywhere I looked. One day, as I leafed through *Paleo Magazine* in the checkout line at the grocery store, the following paragraph, in an article about autoimmune disease, caught my eye:

> Autoimmune disease is a case of mistaken identity: The line between self and non-self becomes blurred. . . . Symptoms are the body's cry for help. Telling you to replace anger with love isn't some soft, New Age philosophy. Studies show that negative emotions increase inflammation, so if you've been mad at

your body for years, it's in your best interest to start practicing forgiveness.

By thinking of autoimmunity as a battle within the self, patients are accepting a metaphor that science handed to them: in the mid-twentieth century, researchers began to describe the immune system as something designed not only to defend against the foreign, but also to tolerate the "self."

On a rainy November day, I met with Warwick Anderson, one of the authors of *Intolerant Bodies*, at the Bowery Hotel in Manhattan. Anderson has a historian's passion for his subject, as well as a historian's caution about what is definitively known. He explained that in 1948 the Australian virologist Frank Macfarlane Burnet, who later received a Nobel Prize for his work, posited that the immune system is fundamentally engaged in distinguishing between self and nonself as a way of learning to "tolerate" the body's own tissue. "Recognition of 'self' from 'not-self' is probably the basis of immunology," Burnet wrote in a 1948 paper.

Burnet introduced a framework that still governs how many researchers think of the immune system and the scientific language of autoimmunity. His fundamental contribution, Anderson told me, was "basically to say, 'The interesting thing is not that the immune system defends the body against the foreign; the interesting thing is that the immune system tolerates the body.'" But along the way, the language of self overtook the language of tolerance. As it happens, Burnet was initially hesitant about the term "self" since it was not a scientific one. But in the end he went with it, Anderson thinks, because he was deeply interested in Freud and the French philosopher Henri Bergson. "If he weren't philosophically minded, he would never have come up with the idea of tolerance of self," Anderson told me. And so it is in some sense an accident of terminology—a coincidence—that immunology uses the word "self" to refer to the body's own tissue, while laypeople use it to refer to the concept of personal identity. After all, another way to describe what happens is simply that the immune system learns to tolerate the body's tissue, distinguishing what is pathogenic from what is nonpathogenic.

In addition, popular culture and medical science alike have come to frame the immune system as a valiant force deployed to protect us. The innate and adaptive branches of the immune system are both characterized, if we are to put it neutrally, by cells that respond to things like pathogens and toxins. For example, macrophages, which are large white blood cells, essentially eat the virus or the toxin they encounter. Scientists have described this action metaphorically as a search-and-destroy mission, in which our immune cells "attack" and "overwhelm" "invading pathogens." This is how most of us now imagine our immunity: as a kind of ethno-nationalist military enterprise, nature's defense system. (I found I couldn't scrub language like "vanquish" and "defend" from these pages.)

The comedian George Carlin, recalling a childhood before the advent of Purell, explores this line of thinking in one of his bits, demonstrating how deeply the analogy has taken root in our minds. His immune system, he tells us, "is equipped with the biological equivalent of fully automatic, military assault rifles with night vision and laser scopes." He goes on:

> When my white blood cells are on patrol, reconnoitering my bloodstream, seeking out strangers and other undesirables, if they see any—any—suspicious-looking germs of any kind, they don't fuck around. They whip out the weapons, wax the motherfucker, and deposit the unlucky fellow directly into my colon! Into my colon! There's no nonsense. There's no Miranda warning, there's none of that three-strikes-and-you're-out shit. First offense, BAM! Into the colon you go.

Like Carlin, we tend to conceive of our immunity as a powerful personalized defense system, or as a "magical and for the most part invisible protective cloak," as the critic Barbara Ehrenreich puts it. That sentimental notion makes us think of it as something ineluctably good. But the immune system also does things like "aiding" cancer cells "to spread and establish new tumors throughout the body," as Ehrenreich notes. Macrophages—the kind of innate immune cell that can ingest pathogens—can be "reeducated" by cancer cells to become "factories" for tumor growth, a 2008 *Scientific American* article reported.

By anthropomorphizing white blood cells (as distinct from, say, liver cells), we reinforce our belief in the special status of the immune system as an intimate defender. When, in autoimmunity, the immune system attacks the body instead of defending it, it feels natural to experience this as a betrayal in which we are both betrayer and betrayed. Metaphors shape how we think, and so if antibodies are soldiers fighting off an incursion of germs, then autoimmune processes become cases of mistaken friendly fire. How *not* to interrogate the psychological implications of that?

What does it matter, you might wonder, how we *think* about the disease we have? But these metaphors had profound implications for me and for the people I interviewed, many of whom saw their illness as a form of personal failure requiring self-indictment.

In this sense, we are misled by metaphor into seeing personal significance where there may be merely accident—or, indeed, systemic causes. It is, in a way, irrational to view the immunological consequence of contracting a virus at a stressful time or your body's reaction to autogenic chemicals at the dry cleaner's you live above as a profound comment about your identity. But this is precisely what the metaphor of self-attack leads many people to do. One might say the same about our tendency to equate autoimmunity and suicide. After all, in cancer it is also the self's own cells that go awry, multiplying uncontrollably—and yet we frame cancer as an other to be battled. By contrast, in some sense we feel as if our antibodies *are* us.

While this confusion has roots in immunology's early vocabulary of selfhood, the idea that disease is a physical expression of a metaphysical condition is not new. It is deeply embedded in Western Judeo-Christian thinking, going back at least to the Christian notion that illness is entangled with sin: "Confess your faults one to another, and pray for one another, that ye may be healed," we read in James 5:16. Christianity saw illness as a sign of spiritual taint—a metaphor for sin. In the Gospel, the sick are healed when they accept faith. Our word "pain" is from the Latin *poena*, or "penalty," later the Old French *peine*, or "suffering," as punishment. In the twentieth century, Freud and his descendants updated this framework by psychologizing illness: the body's symptoms were now not a sign of sin but a sign of taboo or repressed emotions. Still a metaphor.

What is new is that today, in our secular, individualistic nation, an amorphous illness is seen inevitably as an opportunity to uncover the *authentic* nature of the self and improve it, a project squarely in line with other obsessions of our neoliberal society. The focus on personal realization obscures the fact that it is not our *selves* that are wrong but the very structure of our society, with its failing support systems, its poor chemical regulation, its food deserts, its patchwork health care delivery. Autoimmunity is internalized by patients as an opportunity for the ultimate self-management project. But in fact it is a manifestation of a flawed collective project. If it is an indictment of anything, it is an indictment not of our personhood but of our impulse to see social problems as being *about* our personhood, instead of a consequence of our collective shortcomings as co-citizens of this place and time.

THERE ARE OTHER WAYS OF thinking about autoimmunity. In the 1990s, the immunologist Polly Matzinger became concerned that the self/nonself model assumed that the immune system was almost exclusively concerned with foreign matter. She proposed a different model, known as the "danger model," theorizing that the immune system is focused instead on identifying what is *dangerous*. (Her system makes sense of one of the great immunological mysteries, which is why the immune system can tolerate the presence of a fetus; according to her model, it is because the fetus is not dangerous.) Autoimmune disease, Matzinger thinks, happens because the system is set up to respond to chemical distress calls, some of which may come from damaged cells *in* the body rather than from foreign material. In her model, autoimmunity is a consequence not of a battle with the self but of an imprecise biological function, like cell replication gone awry. In this sense, autoimmunity would not be a struggle of self against self but the expression of a body overwhelmed by modern chemicals, viruses, traumas, and a degraded food chain. An expression of a body convinced that danger was all around.

And yet the symbolic suggestiveness of Burnet's immunological nomenclature still shapes how both patients and doctors alike respond to autoimmunity. We continue to describe it as a process in which a body has started attacking its own self. This discourse almost irresistibly makes a patient feel that their own divided emotions about their life shapes their symptoms.

Autoimmunity, then, is awash in the collisions and illogic of modern Western culture. At its heart *is* a conflict—but it is, I contend, a sociopolitical one, not a personal one. The irony is that even as the people I interviewed recognized the sociopolitical dimensions of their condition, they had also internalized the idea, as I had, that something about *them* was the problem, and that it rested on them alone to fix the inauthenticity that made them stressed-out and unhappy. In the United States, there are few autoimmune centers, despite the millions of Americans suffering from autoimmune disease. And there is little political action to regulate chemicals or—despite the work of the Black Lives Matters protests—overcome the structural racism that contributes to the wear and tear on bodies known as "weathering." Rather, suffering and sometimes lonely individuals try on their own to figure out whether gluten, or eggs, or their dry-cleaned clothes are making their symptoms worse. At night the kitchens are full of people like me, cooking a meal for their family, and then a separate one for themselves.

In fact, the idea of autoimmunity as the expression of a conflicted self could be said to serve a purpose that reinforces the societal status quo more than it elucidates biology. First, it gives the patients a story they can focus on and attempt to exert control over. It gives biographical meaning to the disease that otherwise is being described in clinical terms in fifteen-minute appointments by a physician with whom, most likely, the patient has almost no relationship. Instead, the patients tell themselves a story that, painful though it might be, offers them a modicum of control—and the promise of both biological and spiritual healing. In doing so, it makes the illness an individual problem rather than a social issue.

Second—and relatedly—it suggests to the rest of us that these patients are not our problem. The people who brought the disease upon themselves, who were, let's say, *given* to disease, are their own problem. Their illness is personal. If they are stuck in negative thinking, their difficult view of life is for them to overcome—or accede to.

If neurasthenic sensitivity was the hallmark of nineteenth-century invalidism, a kind of hyperpersonalized concern with wellness is the hallmark of twenty-first-century invalidism—a quality that lets the rest of us dismiss the invalid as fussy or oversensitive while we get back to our frenetic, endlessly connected, productive lives. As Bernie S. Siegel, a surgeon who taught at the Yale School of Medicine, wrote in his best-selling *Love, Medicine, and Miracles* (1986), "There are no incurable diseases, only incurable people." It's no coincidence, then, that much of the nation responded to the novel coronavirus along these lines, with many Americans suggesting that those who were at risk—the elderly and people with certain underlying conditions—should just stay home so the rest of America could skip wearing masks, even though such a strategy would have ended up killing even more people than the virus already had.

Who among us doesn't have some inner conflict? And who, when suffering an inexplicable misfortune for the first time, does not ask, "Why me?" When no one can tell you exactly why you're sick, it is surprisingly easy to tell yourself a story about the illness. Why me? *Because* of me. You identify with your illness and feel that somehow you have caused it. "What a grotesque being I am to be sure," wrote Alice James in her diary, drawing a connection between her self and her undiagnosable illness. "Self-disgust" reads the last entry of the extraordinary diary of W. N. P. Barbellion, an English naturalist who died of multiple sclerosis in the early twentieth century and recorded his slow decline. My soul shivered at the dusty sorrow of it.

Then, too, there is the fact—not documented in the medical literature but true of every sick person I have known—that illness causes a sense of apprehension that, before it is recognized as disease, seems psychological, setting the stage for some identification of the mind and body. The writer and editor Norman Cousins, in *Anatomy of an Illness, as Perceived by the Patient*, notes that the night before he got acutely sick with a disabling connective tissue disease, he had flown from Russia to New York. As he drove from the airport to his home in Connecticut, he notes, "I could feel an uneasiness deep in my bones." Unease, dis-ease: Which is which, and does one's unease (or dis-ease) come before the disease or follow upon the pathological processes?

ONE NIGHT I WOKE UP from a dream that I had been with my mother, walking in Brooklyn along a forsythia-lined street, both of us weeping with happiness at seeing each other. I missed her so much it felt like I had a hole in the middle of my body. The orange light of the streetlamp cast an eerie glow through the slats of the blinds in our small bedroom. Jim lay sleeping beside me, his face relaxed. The air-conditioning hummed monotonously.

Which had come first, I wondered—caught up in metaphorical

thinking—my mother's death or my illness? Did the death trigger my illness? Or had I been ill all along, and that was part of why my body cried out for my mother when she died? Had I been the daughter I could have been? The daughter who laughed instead of worried?

I remember, I don't remember. It was true that my illness had gotten worse at the end of the three months of 2008 in which my mother was in and out of the hospital, declining precipitously, confused by tumors that had metastasized in her brain. She lived then in Connecticut with my father and their two dogs, who often lay curled at her feet. For weeks I'd traveled from Brooklyn to Connecticut to help my father take care of her. One day, as I sat beside her on the couch where she rested, she opened her warm brown eyes and said, in a brief moment of clarity, "I just don't want you to spend your life going from hill to hill, Meg. There are other ways to live." She died at the age of fifty-five on Christmas Day 2008; the next morning I ended up in urgent care with a sinus infection. "Poor thing," the clinic doctor in Fairfield said, after examining my ears and nose. "You've let this get really severe. But the antibiotics will clear it up. Get some rest." I took a course of antibiotics, I rested, and I never got better.

It is hard to know what happened when, because for so long I wasn't sure that I was sick. Sometimes I wonder, had I always been sick, since I was a child with aching knees and bouts of exhaustion? Or had I not been sick at all until my family rented a house after my college graduation, close to Lyme, Connecticut, after which my neurological symptoms began? Was life perhaps just a long chronic illness, as a prominent feminist historian would later ask me after I gave a talk about chronic illness—an implication being that it was my identification with my illness that made me "ill"? (Alexander Pope: "This long disease, my life." But Pope, historians think, lived with Pott's disease, or tuberculosis of the spine, from childhood on.)

I don't think it is the case that my mother's death caused my illness. In fact, I know it is not. But I also wonder about the ways that the disappearance of my mother, that bulwark, led to an absence, an ellipsis, into which both dis-ease and disease rushed, unbalancing an equilibrium that had more or less existed until that point. Or think of it this way: I was more run-down when she died than I had ever been. Maybe exhaustion, combined with the virus I caught, was the tipping point, one hit too many to my immune system, after which whatever was already going on snowballed unstoppably downward.

The entanglement of self and sickness became a mirrored distortion, a fun house I feared I was never going to escape, when I realized that I couldn't tell whether my "self" was attacking "myself" without "my" knowledge or influence. Was it true that every time I got stressed about my work or had a fight with Jim "I" was making "myself" sick? Who was "I" and who was "myself," and which had intention, and which didn't? Did intention matter? I was tired, and confused. In my thick fatigue I saw myself reflected as little slivers of biology: a triangle of eye, a shard of thymus, a fragment of viral debris, here, there, and everywhere.

ELEVEN

MIND/BODY

Whatever I told myself about internal conflicts and illness, there was one thing I did begin to pay serious attention to: the role stress played in my life. The science I was reading suggested just how harmful continual stress could be. This wasn't the episodic premodern stress of a human racing away from a lion (as the books' authors always seemed to point out), but a continual grind of daily life that wore down resilience and could do real damage to the body.

Before I encountered the science, though, I encountered the slightly degraded popularization of it: in the view of some of the more alternative practitioners I saw, my disease was brought on at least partly by ambition, which caused me to work too much. No one said this in so many words, but they suggested that I "pushed myself too hard" and experienced "too much stress," taxing my adrenals and leading to a compromised immune system. A nutritionist told me to stop ignoring the "part of myself that needed nurturing." A physiotherapist I saw proposed that the reason I had an injury in my *right* hip was that the right side was the "masculine" side—the side, as she put it, of grand endeavor. She handed me a printout of the chakras and encouraged me to "send energy earthward." An acupuncturist suggested, "Maybe try not to think so much."

In the past, I would have felt these suggestions were New Age jargon; the last one smacked of the recommendations given to Alice James and other nineteenth-century "hysterics" from doctors who thought that mental exertion took too much energy away from women's wombs, thereby enervating them. But I took the counsel to heart, because there was common sense in the message. Sleeping well, relaxing, eating whole foods—I could see how years of stress, poor sleep, and erratic diet could mean that eventually even a healthy body would start to show signs of exhaustion.

Now I turned down work, ensured that I went to sleep early, and in general tried to embrace a new self, a nurturing, relaxed person I have never really been. I *was* starting to see that my life of constant work and worry was a choice, an anchor to which I chained myself. (A friend wrote advising me to take it easy. I replied, "I am strenuously following your advice," and he pointed out that the "strenuously" part might defeat the purpose.) I still flinched whenever anyone suggested I was somehow *responsible* for my disease. I couldn't help hearing, even in the more tactful efforts, the speakers' own need to lie to themselves, to reassure themselves that they would not get sick randomly the way I had, because they were not as tightly wound/stressed/you-name-it as I was. Whatever role stress might play in my illness, I strongly suspected it had not *caused* it. And yet I, too, wanted to imagine that there was a magical solution: that behavioral modifications would lead—voilà—to physical and spiritual wholeness of a sort I'd never experienced before.

That may sound naïve. But I kept going back to the science. Studies show that cortisol levels spike when we answer email and check our phones; endless connectivity takes its toll. More of us inhabit cities or population-dense areas than ever before, too, where traffic has steadily increased. Sleep deprivation can impair functioning as much as alcohol consumption. People who have been awake seventeen hours are the functional equivalent of people with a near DUI level of alcohol intoxication. When you are chronically sleep deprived, inflammation and illness creep in. Loud sounds arouse parts of our brains connected to fear, which in turn trigger a spike in blood pressure and stress hormones like cortisol. The World Health Organization recommends a maximum threshold of forty decibels at night for healthy sleep—a threshold that is exceeded by a single truck braking on the street.

Many of us have felt the need to take a break from the chaos of our daily lives for our health's sake. The world becomes more stressful by the day: constant inputs, tedious bureaucratic tasks or requests, emails, text messages. Indeed, a desire for less stimulation has been afflicting Americans at least since the invention of the steam engine. Concerned about "the thousand intricate problems . . . which perplex those who struggle to-day in our teeming city hives," the neurologist Silas Weir Mitchell wondered, "Have we lived too fast?" He published *Wear and Tear; or, Hints for the Overworked* not in 2021, but in 1871. Mitchell is one of the men responsible for diagnosing an epidemic of hysteria and neurasthenia among nineteenth-century Americans brought on by the stimulation of modern life, which was overtaxing their nerves.

The contemporary version of the notion that stress shapes health was first floated by two men in the early twentieth century. The first, Walter B. Cannon, was a Harvard physiologist who demonstrated that emotions could affect the body's physiology. Before his discovery, he was using the new technology of X-rays to study peristalsis—the intestinal contractions that push waste out of our bodies—in animals. He noticed that when the animals were fighting or distressed, peristalsis slowed down. Drawing their blood, he found that it contained elevated amounts of what we now call "epinephrine" or "adrenaline," a hormone secreted by the adrenal gland near the kidney. Faced with the evidence that emotions had changed the animal's physiology, he performed a follow-up experiment that led him to two key medical ideas. The first is the famous fight-or-flight response. Cannon noted that, faced with danger, the body slows digestion (because it takes energy away from our muscles) and produces hormones like epinephrine to give us the best possible chance of outrunning a predator. The second is the modern version of the idea that the body will return to a stable baseline after the perceived threat is gone, a process he called "homeostasis." In 1936, Cannon gave a lecture exhorting medical clinicians to see that they were facing a new kind of American illness: modernity's disruption of homeostasis. Where "plagues and pestilence" once killed most people, now it was the "strains and stresses" of modern life making people sick by disrupting homeostasis. "Chronic emotional upset," intensified by the fast pace of modern life, was the new source of illness.

If Cannon was the first to use the term "stress," a Hungarian doctor named Hans Selye popularized the word in the sense we use it today, after discovering that stress can suppress the immune system. As a young professor, Selye worked on endocrinology, or the way hormones communicate in the body. To study their effects, he embarked on an experiment that involved injecting lab rats with an ovarian extract. But as Robert M. Sapolsky notes in *Why Zebras Don't Get Ulcers*, Selye was so awkward in the lab that the rats kept escaping, forcing him to chase them around the room before he could catch and inject them. At the end of the study, Selye found that the rats had an unusual number of peptic ulcers, enlarged adrenal glands, and "shrunken immune tissue." At first, he thought this was because of the ovarian extract he had injected. But when he ran a control group of rats injected with a saline solution, he found that these rats *also* ended up with an unusual number of peptic ulcers, enlarged adrenal glands, and shrunken immune tissue. Reflecting on the finding, he realized that alarm—the distress caused by being chased around the room by a klutzy professor—might have made the animals sick, and he designed a new experiment to identify whether his thesis was correct. It was.

To describe the process that led to the animals' disease, Selye used the term "stress" and what he called "the general adaptation syndrome" to codify the response the body has to stressors. (We now call it the "stress response.") In his pioneering work, he suggested that not only do emotional demands on the body cause stress, but also that, if the stress is ongoing, it can contribute to hormonal dysregulation and a variety of other problems, from allergic reactions to ulcers and high blood pressure and kidney disease. The stress response is an adaptive function to help us survive periodic danger, flooding our body with the extra oxygen to help us flee the proverbial lion. But it is maladaptive for Westerners: our bodies were not designed to feel stress routinely, as we do dealing with any assortment of pressures that modern life has brought with it. When stress becomes constant, Selye showed, it stops helping us and starts hurting us.

Today, the idea that chronic stress makes us ill—that our thoughts and experiences can, in a scientifically plausible way, alter our physiology to the point of introducing disease—is an accepted one. Chronic stress releases continual jolts of stress hormones, which can raise blood pressure and cause cardiovascular disease, leading to a hardening of the arteries. It makes gut-related illnesses like irritable bowel syndrome worse. And it can lead to dysfunction in cortisol production.

Increasingly, it's becoming evident that stress can play a role in autoimmune and other immune-related illnesses, too. Recently, scientists discovered that they had overlooked a key step in the stress response: in the first half hour or so following a stressor, the body's immune system becomes *more* active. This makes evolutionary sense—the body is preparing for a wound or possible infection, say. Then, over the following hours, the body typically tries to return immune activity to a baseline, by releasing steroid hormones to inhibit white blood cell production. But some people get stuck in the heightened state, with an overactive immune system. For these people, as Sapolsky observes, "repeated ups and downs ratchet the system upward, biasing it toward autoimmunity." Research shows that some people with rheumatoid arthritis, for example, have immune cells that are insufficiently responsive to the rising steroid levels that are supposed to dampen their activity. The repetitions of ongoing stressors elevate the risk that "something uncoordinated occurs," as Sapolsky puts it, leaving the immune system more likely to attack the wrong targets and the patient more symptomatic.

It may make sense, then, that many autoimmune patients—me included—have reported that stressful periods lead to a worsening of their symptoms. When I was most ill, I had noted that just *anticipating* a stressful occasion seemed to lead to my waking up sick the day of a big event or a hectic schedule full of things I didn't entirely want to do, which contributed to my worry that my sickness might really be psychosomatic. But reading about the mechanics of stress offered a possible explanation for why this occurred. For example, Sapolsky points out that the human body responds to anticipated and imagined stress *as if* it is lived stress. This capacity for imagining and anticipating makes stress damaging. Our subconscious takes our conscious fears seriously, and adjusts our biology accordingly.

Learning about the way humans respond to stress assuaged one fear, but it set off another. Running to catch the bus on DeKalb Avenue, my hair wet, my coat unbuttoned, anxious to make it to an appointment, I'd suddenly think, *Oh no! I'm stressed!* I'd stop and take gulps of cold air, cortisol speeding through my body, my heart pounding. Soon the stress of trying *not* to be stressed was wearing me out, winding me into an anxious, coiled state. One night, I was telling Jim about some of the things I was learning—the way stress does seem to alter the immune system, when he said, "This seems like one of the hardest things about being sick in the way you're sick: being sick makes you stressed. But being stressed makes you sicker."

That night I couldn't stop turning over his words. I knew that unpredictability and lack of control make people more stressed: studies show that people in pain who can control their own pain medication use much less of it than when nurses control the meds. And here I was, sick and without any control. I had no name for what was wrong with me, no possibility of treatment, and no sense of why my symptoms were happening when they did. I was in a perpetual stress state because I had a stress-inducing illness, with episodic, amorphous, migrating pain, and total uncertainty about what caused it. Like others in this situation, I couldn't do anything about my illness or even know when to do things about it. The illness *responded* to stress, but at the same time the illness *was* a state of perpetual stress, weighing on me like a boulder. Which is one reason people hunger for a clear diagnosis.

Once I understood the profound biological feedback loops of stress, I could not avoid reflecting, too, on all the ways that America's lack of a social safety net and its history of systemic racism make people sicker, on top of everything else. This is the theory of Arline T. Geronimus, a public health researcher who in 1992 coined the "weathering hypothesis" to explain why so many young Black women have more health issues—and poorer maternal outcomes—than their well-off white peers. The weathering hypothesis theorizes that African American women have more illness in early adulthood as a result of the constant stress of systemic racism and, for some, the challenges of facing socioeconomic disadvantages. Further research suggests that socioeconomic disadvantages and structural insecurity lead to telomere shortening—a key measure of aging—and a higher allostatic load (wear and tear caused by stress). While conservatives like to put the focus for health on individual responsibility and "lifestyle," a term they use as a weapon, Geronimus's research reminds us of the social, interconnected nature of our bodies and our health, and the way that racism exacts debilitating vigilance from Black bodies. That vigilance has an invisible physical cost. The calamity here is not one of personal failure but of societal failure: the conditions of insecurity that systemic racism not only perpetuates but actively fosters. The state of a person's immune system is, among other things, a reflection of that person's socioeconomic status and their history as a citizen of a flawed polis, I now understood.

TWELVE

POSITIVE THINKING

The counterpart of the notion that stress makes us ill is the idea that positive thinking can heal us. In 1979, when Norman Cousins published *Anatomy of an Illness, as Perceived by the Patient,* he chronicled a self-prescribed "laughing cure" he had embarked on. Newly diagnosed with ankylosing spondylitis, in which the joints of the spine fuse together, he had been told to get his affairs in order. Instead, he embarked on a complex, all-natural recovery plan. Tired of staying in the hospital, where the nutrition was not ideal ("What seemed inexcusable to me was the profusion of processed foods, some of which contained preservatives or harmful dyes"), he moved to a hotel. Instead of taking painkillers, he persuaded his physician to let him take large doses of vitamin C. Instead of worry, he decided to manipulate his own body chemistry by purposefully achieving a sustained emotional state of delight—a laughing cure.

When I read Cousins's book, I thought, *Why not try a little laughter?* I made a plan to "have fun." Like Cousins, I watched comic movies in hopes of healing myself. I sat on the couch, ready to laugh at

Will Ferrell or Maya Rudolph. I talked on the phone to friends. I took long hot baths. I did relax for a while, only to get anxious about all the emails I had to answer, the books I wasn't writing because I was watching TV. I disliked my sense of being out of time, by which I meant, I now see, the sense of being out of *productive* time, unable to contribute to the sheer volume of engagement and connectivity that characterizes the contemporary workday. By two p.m. I'd be looking at my watch every few minutes, wondering how much time had passed, eager to try to get some work done. (Time doesn't fly when you're *trying* to have fun.)

Don't go from hill to hill, Meg, my mother would have said.

Why had I not absorbed that lesson? Why could I not? If she were here, I thought, I would leap at the chance to drop everything to spend time with her. I sat at my window, looking into our backyard, the pagan green explosion of leaves, the defiant flame of the Japanese maple, lost in the smoky distance until the doorbell rang: a delivery of school supplies for our downstairs neighbor. I wanted to be the one eagerly opening the packages of pencils and notebooks, inhaling the scent of fresh starts. The truth was, I was lucky to do work—writing—that really was pleasure. Writing was the way I knew myself: as someone who searched for the sounds of meaning, who thought my way through distress on the page. Instead, I was locked in a fragile pursuit of someone else's idea of fun.

THE LATEST WAVE OF BELIEF in positive thinking dates to the 1970s, when a handful of studies suggested that positive thinking was beneficial to the resilience of cancer patients. People began to assume that "healing ties" or having a "fighting spirit" were determinants of cancer outcomes. In a landmark study, the Stanford psychiatrist David Spiegel found that women with metastatic breast cancer who had gotten support from group sessions had "lower mood-disturbance . . . and were less phobic." They also appeared to live longer than the women in the control group—twice as long on average, or 36.6 months compared to 18.9 months.

Spiegel had been skeptical when he set out, expecting to uncover evidence that positive thinking did not work, but he embraced his findings—and so did America. Today, the notion that a positive attitude helps cure us can be found everywhere. On *CBS Sunday Morning* in 2004, Lance Armstrong announced, of his triumph over advanced testicular cancer, "You can't deny the fact that a person with a positive and optimistic attitude does a lot better." Mark Herzlich, a former linebacker for the New York Giants, has said publicly that his positive attitude helped him overcome bone cancer. The "pinkwashing" of breast cancer means we usually hear from breast cancer survivors who cheerlead about positive mindsets, as Anne Boyer notes in *The Undying*.

Positive thinking in the face of illness purports to give us back a modicum of control. It suggests coherence in a chaotic world. It makes willpower and mindset meaningful again—even though willpower is one of the things that disease can prove to be a false (or at least overdetermined) construct. No wonder so many Americans still believe that positive thinking has a role to play in health. I, too, wished that it could lift me from my morass of sickness, even as I instinctively distrusted our cultural embrace of it: the American affection for positive thinking reflects a desire for illness stories to have neat resolutions and uplifting moral outcomes. Busy trying to follow in Cousins's footsteps, I found that the burden of positivity weighed on me after just a few days. What was I supposed to do with my fears, my darker thoughts? Tamp them down? Pretend I couldn't taste the metallic tang of terror? How was I supposed to be positive about the amorphous and never-ending exhaustion, the sense that my mitochondria were off-kilter? I loved my friends; I wanted my life back. Wasn't that positive enough?

In the aftermath of Spiegel's finding, numerous studies, including a follow-up he conducted in 2007, have failed to replicate his results or show a connection between optimism and disease outcomes in cancer. In one of the most rigorous, James Coyne, a professor of psychology at the University of Pennsylvania, studied nearly eleven hundred people with cancer and found no correlation among optimism, positive thinking, and cancer survival rates. Since then, most studies have suggested that positive thinking does not lead to better outcomes with breast cancer.

WHILE POSITIVE THINKING WAS TOO reductive a notion for me to embrace, I was startled to read about evidence that the brain (or mind) and the immune system are engaged in an especially deep and complex dialogue, one that can be affected by thoughts, mindset, and psychological "primes" in ways that we are still learning about.

I had assumed that the immune system busily fights off infections all by itself, an independent contractor, having absorbed the scientific dogma that the nervous system and the immune system had little to do with each other. But when I began researching the mind-body connection, I came across the quickly growing field of psychoneuroimmunology, which looks at how thoughts and unconscious priming *do* influence immune expression in ways that go far beyond the effects of stress. Research has identified a profound connection—and ongoing communication—between the two systems, one that in some ways has reshaped how scientists think.

In 1974, Robert Ader, a psychologist at the University of Rochester, conducted an experiment about behavioral conditioning using rats with the immunologist Nicholas Cohen, and found that our brain could powerfully influence our immune system. The discovery was a fortuitous accident. Ader's experiment was originally designed to to see if the rats would develop an aversion to a saccharin solution (which they usually love) if he gave them a nausea-inducing immunosuppressive drug, cyclophosphamide, with it. And, as expected, the rats did become averse to the water: they didn't want to drink it even when it was unaccompanied by the drug.

The surprising thing was what happened next. Ader continued to give the rats saccharin solution *without* the drug in order to see how long the aversion would last. And he found that many of these rats, unexpectedly, got sick—some even died. The rats in the control group did not.

In other words, when the rats drank the plain saccharin water, their immune systems reacted as if the drug were being given to them even though it wasn't, simply because their brain had been conditioned to associate the solution with immune suppression. Ader and Cohen then ran a second experiment, designed to make sure the first result was not luck. They found the same result. A mental association was weakening the rats' immune system even though they were no longer receiving the actual immune-dampening drug itself. In the paper describing their work, Ader and Cohen concluded that "there may be an intimate and virtually unexplored relationship between the central nervous system and immunologic processes."

This discovery helped usher in a new way of thinking about the brain–immune system connection. Some of the most fascinating experiments have been overseen by Ellen Langer, a professor of psychology at Harvard who works on aging and illness. In her work, Langer is interested in the idea, as *The New York Times* put it, that "what people needed to heal themselves was a psychological 'prime'—something that triggered the body to take curative measures all by itself." Langer has demonstrated that our immune systems respond to all sorts of unconscious cues. In one landmark experiment, which she calls a "counterclockwise" study, she monitored two groups of aging men. In one group, the men were encouraged to view themselves as twenty years younger than they were, listening to music of an earlier era and speaking about news of the era in the present tense. (They were also treated as if they were younger.) At the end of one week, the men's sight and hearing had improved, they were stronger, and they had more energy. "It sounded like Lourdes," she told *The New York Times*.

One gray Saturday morning, the sky smudged by clouds, I spoke with Langer by phone. It was one of the most challenging conversations I have ever had, in the way that it invited me to think outside of known dichotomies while also resisting the sloppier aspects of the embrace of positive thinking. If I had spent years trying to disentangle mind and body, the conversation with Langer in some ways upended my resistance to the idea that they could be connected. In fact, it reminded me of what the poet in me already knew: thoughts are, in a sense, somatic. The question is what we do with that idea, and how we use it in the face of all that is uncertain about our health and our bodies.

Langer grew interested in the mind-body relationship in the 1970s, when her mother was diagnosed with metastatic breast cancer. Langer, then twenty-nine, refused to let anyone who was not "uplifting," as she put it, see her mother. A few weeks later, when the doctors reexamined her mother, the cancer was gone. The oncologist wanted to write it up as a "medical mystery," but, as she told me, "There was nothing medical about that." Since then, she has studied how outlook and expectation shape health, with astonishing results, discovering that our thoughts can change our health—but only if we really *believe* the thoughts. For example, she conducted a study based on the popular idea that pilots have excellent vision. Langer found that people's vision improved if they thought they were in an airplane simulator. If they did the same activity, but the simulator was broken, nothing changed. Likewise, in another study, she studied the blood sugar level of diabetic patients and found that it rose and fell according to how they were *experiencing* time, not according to actual time, a finding with startling impact for the management of type 2 diabetes. The key here is that simply imagining an outcome does not appear to change much. But when we *feel* something in an embodied way, measurable change may occur.

As we talked, Langer underscored that she is not saying that people who die from cancer are to blame for their own illness or can decide to cure themselves overnight. But she came close to saying that perhaps—

given the right tools—we can heal ourselves almost instantaneously. Because she knows we live in a relentlessly biomedical world, she is interested in finding ways to determine "how we can apply our mental capacities to increase control of our health and well-being." In her work she does this through mindfulness, teaching people how to mind "differently," she explained to me. "I smashed my ankle many years ago," she told me. "The doctor said I'd never walk without a limp. The problem is I forgot about it; now I have no limp."

In some ways, Langer is a realist: she tries to get people to notice which underlying realities, from environment to mood, make their illness worse and to manage those triggers. "If you stand in a barn for half an hour and your hay fever gets worse, I would suggest you avoid the barn," she said drily. (She does not suggest that you go in the barn and tell yourself you feel fine.) But she also believes that actively reorienting our attitude to overcome social and cultural cues is important.

I asked her about my case, explaining that how I felt changed day by day. First, she graciously acknowledged the reality of my symptoms. Then she explained that with a disease like mine, which ebbs and flares, "if some days are fine, I would ask people first, what is the difference between days you are fine and days you are not fine? If you sometimes feel good, it means you don't have the disease all the time. Why is that, and how can you get to inhabit that 'not all the time' more frequently?"

Some devotees of mind-body practices reduce the complex role of the mind's influence on the body to a simpler one than Langer assigns it. In fact, it seems that most people fall into one of two camps: they tend either to reject the role of the mind entirely or to embrace it so fully they erase the obdurate reality of the body. What I liked about Langer was the way she made room for mystery and clarified that if thoughts have any role in modulating illness, it isn't a simple one.

Of course, what we *expect* to feel plays a role in what we do feel. Nortin Hadler, an emeritus professor of medicine at UNC–Chapel Hill, talks about the consequences of so-called negative labeling: evidence shows that when you give patients a diagnosis, they tend to feel sicker or more vulnerable than they did without one. Focusing on symptoms, studies suggest, can make those symptoms seem more severe. Distracting yourself from your own worst thoughts about your condition, this research suggests, can be genuinely helpful. I found that in my own suffering this technique worked great for pain. But it didn't help with the dizziness, brain fog, and neurological problems I was having.

Illness goes far beyond the mind, of course—an idea that the positive thinking model wants to deny. "The flip side of positivity is . . . a harsh insistence on personal responsibility." So says Barbara Ehrenreich in *Bright-Sided: How Positive Thinking Is Undermining America.* That insistence led to decades of self-help books and scores of alternative medicine practitioners suggesting that cancer was a disease of repressed stress. (One mother of a son with cancer told David Spiegel, the researcher who had done the famous study about positive thinking, that her support group urged her to accept that he was sick because he was "unloved.") This line of thought was so pervasive that as late as 1989 the mayor of Princeton, diagnosed with a metastatic melanoma of the eye, considered it necessary to write an op-ed explaining that *she* was not responsible for her cancer. "Cancer cells are internalized anger gone on a field trip all over our bodies," she stated, summarizing the alt-medical idea. "Give me a break." The problem with this framework, she explained, is that it robbed her of the dignity of her actual struggle with illness: "If I die, I don't want to feel like a failure. My doctor tells me I've embarked on an unknown trail; he doesn't know of anyone else with eye melanoma who has undergone this particular chemotherapy. It's scary; I want the dignity of that reality."

The dignity of that reality. I didn't believe my illness was psychosomatic, nor did I want to make others feel theirs was. But like any good poet, I suppose, I was drawn to those who were thinking about the intertwined relationship between mind and body, those scientists who genuinely wanted to understand more about the relationship between the immune system and the nervous system. I found Langer's approach refreshing for its openness. It connected to my own lived sense that my illness, which I firmly believed had some cause other than my mind, responded to lifestyle intervention and modifications in a way that Western biomedicine still had little to say about. I craved a more nuanced discourse of the mind and the body: after all, the idea that thoughts could influence body and body could influence thought hardly seems surprising. The problem is that so many patients' ailments have been reduced to one or the other as a way of shutting down inquiry.

To have the dignity of one's reality: this, I realized, was why I worked so hard to find language to tell my story. I wanted to show how the emphasis on the psychological nature of chronic illness in a culture that pathologizes the failure to "overcome" robbed people of grace, while instructing them to suffer their illness *with* grace.

THIRTEEN

POSSIBILITY

In August 2013, I published an article about my experience of getting sick with an autoimmune disease, in which I talked about the symptoms my doctors had been unable to account for. Afterward, I got letters from people around the country. Some suggested that my illness was due to the mercury fillings in my teeth (it was true I had an almost comical amount of them). Others thought that it was the wi-fi router, poisoning me with electromagnetic radiation. A man from upstate New York suggested that my "second heart"—a long-ignored organ supposedly positioned behind the knee—wasn't working, and offered, for the modest fee of a thousand dollars, to come to my house with a machine of his devising that would allow me to get second-heart assistance. A pacemaker for the lymphatic system, as he put it. Another woman suggested I come try something she called "the Mortdecai machine," which would restore my spiritual energies and therefore my body. The suggestions were mostly nutty. But in the middle of the night, I woke up anxious. Could it in fact be the case that I had a deficient second heart? Might my router be making me sick? Did I need to reorient my whole understanding of how the world worked, like Neo in *The Matrix*, choosing the red pill?

Then several people wrote in explaining that they believed I had Lyme disease. My electric shocks and neurological issues, they wrote, were classic symptoms of the infection. *Could they be right?* I wondered. Although I grew up in New York City, my family liked to camp, and we spent the warm summer months in Vermont and on Cape Cod, which, I knew, had some of the highest rates of Lyme disease in the country. My mother used to check us for the bull's-eye rash every day. She had removed many ticks from me when I was a child, but the understanding in those days was that if there was no rash, there was no infection, and I couldn't remember having ever gotten the distinctive bull's-eye rash. After my parents had moved to southeastern Connecticut, their golden retriever had gotten Lyme disease numerous times since they'd moved. The spring after my mother died, I had a circular rash on my torso that persisted for a few weeks, though it never changed in size, as Lyme rashes usually do.

I had of course been tested for the tick-borne infection once, by the bicycle-riding integrative doctor—with negative results. It led me to dismiss the possibility. But an investment banker whom I'd gone to college with wrote to me after reading my piece to tell me that he had tested negative for Lyme disease for months before testing positive and entering treatment, with dramatic results: he went from bedridden to well in just months. I began to wonder if I needed to get retested.

I ENDED UP FINDING the person who would test me in a roundabout way. Early in my online reading about chronic illness, I'd stumbled across a functional medicine practitioner I'll call Matt Galen and decided he could perhaps help me—but he had a long wait list. He had become interested in health after he traveled the world in his twenties and contracted a mysterious illness. After visiting doctors and getting no answers, he started studying medicine and working with healers. Eventually, he got better and opened a functional medicine practice. He was one of these names you came across a lot in the chronic illness community, representative of a new kind of health leadership, consisting largely of men who built online cultish followings around their devotion to the Paleo diet, their dedication to physical self-improvement, and their willingness to synthesize the often-conflicting science of nutrition. Fascinated by the collision of cutting-edge science with borderline obsessiveness, I had lost many hours on their websites, reading about circadian rhythms and the suprachiasmatic nucleus (or so-called master clock). Amid all the conflicting and often dubious information I found online, Galen's newsletter stood out for its rigor. I liked that he was skeptical and evidence based (for example, willing to debunk the idea I often saw on my online patient groups that the additive magnesium stearate was bad for you). Frustrated that my Western doctors hadn't found any answers, and uncertain how much to trust some of the integrative doctors I saw, I put myself on a wait list to meet with Galen remotely. I didn't expect that he would figure out what was wrong with me, but I thought that he might well give me some tips on how to cope and where to look next.

We finally spoke by phone one summer afternoon. I had been feeling slightly better, as I always did in the summer. But the fatigue and brain fog were still challenging. Jim and I were in Greenport again, having rented a friend's house while she was away. She was a poetry editor and a writer. Bookcases stacked with poetry collections lined the walls of the study where I liked to sit in the morning to try to work. The room had a Dutch door facing the front yard, and I would open the top half and let a warm ocean breeze in. Now I listened to Galen go over my labs (low vitamin D, low iron, a positive ANA, and anemia) as my eyes wandered over the beautiful books on my friend's shelves, books of the sort I wanted the chance to write. But I needed my brain to work first. Galen suggested recommitting to the autoimmune Paleo diet; taking a higher-quality glutathione supplement; switching my probiotics to a soil-based brand, closer to what I would have been eating in an earlier era; and being aggressive about getting my vitamin D levels up, because low vitamin D correlates to higher levels of autoimmunity and inflammation, and mounting evidence suggests that vitamin D has an immunomodulatory effect. He advocated doing these things one at a time, so I could keep a record of how each change affected me.

His main recommendation, though, was that for my pain and inflammation I try something called "low-dose naltrexone" (LDN), which I'd read about on message boards. Naltrexone is a drug that blocks opioid receptors and is typically used to help manage alcohol and opioid addiction. Some doctors, though, have found it helpful in very low doses for conditions characterized by immunological dysfunction, including chronic pain. In blocking the opioid receptors, it also blocks endorphin production for a few hours, which leads your body to think you need to make more endorphins. Apparently—or so the advocates claim—a boost of endorphins can help modulate your immune system, though the treatment is still experimental. (LDN is now used by Weill Cornell Medicine in New York City for pain management.) Galen was not an MD, so he was not licensed to prescribe LDN, but he gave me instructions about how to go about getting it. There was a group of people on Yahoo who shared the names of doctors who prescribed it in this off-label way. (Joining this group, I felt like I was getting a code to an inner sanctum of the ill.)

A few days after our call, I made an appointment with an infectious disease doctor who prescribes LDN, whom I'll call Dr. C. Her website proclaimed the importance of listening to patients in order to "hear the diagnosis."

I went to see Dr. C on a late summer day in 2013 that managed to be both humid and slightly cool, leaving me sweating and chilled by the time I hurried from the subway to her building. Her office was appealingly disorganized. A fat dachshund slept curled in the corner, lazily opening his eyes at me. Outside the window was a lush courtyard garden. "I hope you don't mind," Dr. C said, gesturing at the dog. "He has thyroid disease so he's tired. I like to keep him close." I looked more closely at the dog and I could see it—the drooping glaze in his eyes, the puffiness around his facial bones. *Oh god, that's me,* I thought. I suddenly felt a pang of sorrow.

Dr. C spent an hour patiently listening to my history and taking notes on her computer, an old IBM. She asked me about the fact that I dyed my hair—did my symptoms get worse afterward?—and about my stress levels, and then examined me more thoroughly than any doctor had done to date. She noted that because of my jaw structure—I had a narrow palate—I might have a bit of sleep apnea. Perhaps that was one reason I was tired. I liked her; she was extremely precise and knowledgeable, and yet she was patient, too. When I asked halting questions, she took the time to explain the answers in depth.

Based on my previous blood work, she said, she felt comfortable prescribing me LDN. She also wanted to test me for a range of infectious diseases, since I had begun feeling worse after getting that rash in Vietnam, and because I had grown up on the East Coast, camping and hiking in places where Lyme disease is common. She thought we should in fact order not one but several Lyme-disease tests, from different labs. I told her I'd never gotten the classic bull's-eye rash. She said not everyone did and asked me to come back in three weeks, when the lab results would be in.

The LDN came in a little plastic applicator that reminded me of a roll-on deodorant. I was supposed to rub it on my inner arm before bed. Our bodies typically produce the most endorphins late at night. Suppressing their production during these key hours would lead to higher production the next day, theoretically helping me feel better, since endorphins act on opiate receptors in the brain and produce feelings of well-being, along with offering immune-modulating benefits. But, the doctor warned before I left, suppressing nighttime endorphins can have the short-term side effect of creating oddly intense dreams.

Later that week I had a vivid nightmare about a series of terrorist attacks in Brooklyn, as if I were reliving the events of September 11. In this dream, as I had in life, I ran from my house to try to find my family, who worked in Brooklyn Heights, as small pieces of burning paper fell on the ground. But in the dream a flotilla of purple-gray planes hung like plums in the sky, orange rocket smoke streaking the horizon, while I tried to reach my mother and father, struggling through thronging crowds on the narrow cobblestone streets, unable to get to where I was trying to go.

OVER LABOR DAY WEEKEND, I went to the U.S. Open with some friends, one of whom had a bad cold. We sat high up in the arena, talking about our summers. Halfway through the day a group leaving offered us their near-courtside seats to watch Serena and Venus Williams play doubles. We moved down and spread out, enjoying the match. My friend Amanda asked if Jim and I were still trying to have a baby. I was feeling well enough at summer's end to think perhaps I could. I imagined being well, writing, hearing the voices of small children in the next room. It gave me a sense of hope.

Three days later, I had caught my friend's cold. It landed me in bed for two weeks, draining me like a phone running too many apps.

That month, things went steadily downhill.

The LDN was not the magic bullet for me that it had been for others I knew, though I did notice that I had an endorphin rush one day after taking a walk. My thyroid hormones did not return to normal, as some patients' did. In fact, I felt steadily worse. Exhaustion consumed my body. The fatigue was itself fatiguing. I woke early every morning in pain, unable to go back to sleep. Before I opened my eyes, I did a kind of mental check to see if the pain was there. It is hard to describe without using the usual words: I had a headache, achiness, flu-like symptoms. But it's one thing to have these symptoms for a day, or even a week. Suffered daily, they take on a meaning beyond the pain, like being shadowed by a specter. You have a feeling something in your body is trying to defeat you, that something inside you wants you dead. One bright morning I woke and felt joy—the fog is not there!—only for it to jostle through me when I sat up.

The first hours of being awake were so awful that I had to devise strategies for enduring them. In the dark of five a.m., I would make a matcha latte on the recommendation of one of my nutritionists, slowly stirring the vivid green powder into almond milk, and then I would sit very still on the white couch in my living room, waiting for the sun to come up and for the pain to dissipate. I tried to read, but I was too tired to. Sometimes I listened to the radio to feel less alone or looked at recipes I might one day be well enough to make. Other times I lay there and tried to remember, in intricate detail, trips I'd taken in a former life: the cabin in Vermont by the meadow of wildflowers with the winding creek my brother and I waded in; the covered bridge we'd jump from into the Battenkill, the water so cold it shocked the body into a pure wakefulness.

I felt both a resignation that verged on despair and a conviction that somehow my plight could change. If only I could figure out the difference between the good days and the bad days, as Ellen Langer suggested, perhaps I could reverse the disease, or improve.

WHEN I RETURNED TO DR. C's office later that fall to go over the test results, I got some surprising news. First, my doctor said, "You have an extremely high inflammatory marker, here," pointing to one immunological finding, which could be indicative of infection. I also had active Epstein-Barr once again.

"But there's something more significant," she said. Dr. C then showed me contradictory results from three labs that test for Lyme disease—one was negative, while two others were partially positive. I was confused.

"What does this mean?" I asked.

Dr. C explained that the tests could be unreliable because they measure for antibodies to Lyme rather than actual bacteria. Sometimes they picked up autoimmune antibodies instead. In this case, the tests had found some evidence of antibodies to an outer surface protein of the bacterium itself. "You probably have Lyme disease—your symptoms and your blood work suggest it," she continued. But she said she didn't want to prescribe antibiotics—the usual course of treatment for Lyme—because she thought I was so sick that they might harm me.

Instead, she suggested I continue the LDN, take fish oil and apple cider vinegar to help with the inflammation (and some protein malabsorption), and try a phosphatidylcholine drip—a therapy that some integrative doctors use to treat infections. If that didn't work, we could check back in.

After fifteen years in the dark—if I counted from my first bouts of electric shocks and poor health—I at last had a possible name for my remaining problems. Yet instead of feeling relief, I felt I had woken into a nightmare. I wasn't sure whether the disease I had really was untreated Lyme. And even if I did have Lyme disease, there was little agreement about how to treat a patient like me, whose test results were equivocal and who had been diagnosed very late in the course of the infection. Tidy evidence-based protocols were nowhere in sight. Many doctors did not advise antibiotics in such cases. Those who did tended to prescribe months to years of oral and IV antibiotics, which can be dangerous, without clear evidence that such treatment worked. Online, I read posts by people who, even after such treatments, continued to experience debilitating exhaustion and memory impairment or were so disoriented that they had trouble finding their own homes. The stories were not encouraging. So the test results quickly plunged me deeper into uncertainty. This was a diagnosis that posed more questions; the one thing everyone seemed to agree on was that the usual three weeks of antibiotics simply didn't work for patients with late-stage Lyme.

And so embracing the Lyme diagnosis seemed a risky path to walk down. One acquaintance of mine who was similarly diagnosed after years of being ill was on her fifth or sixth course of IV drugs because that was the only treatment she'd found that kept her cognitive faculties functioning. Because evidence on the efficacy of such treatment is mixed, many people believe that "Lyme specialists" are simply preying on vulnerable patients who likely have something else wrong with them that hasn't yet been identified. Then, too, I had spent years learning about how damaging antibiotics were to the body, absorbing the evidence that they played a powerful role in altering the microbiome and contributing to autoimmune diseases. And who knew if I *had* Lyme? Dr. C herself had cautioned that the label "Lyme disease" was easy to pin on a patient's symptoms because the tests can be inaccurate. I understood. I'd gotten my hopes up before. My experience of medicine had led me to conclude that specialists often saw my troubles through their particular lens: An autoimmune disease! A viral issue! Your mind!

In the absence of medical clarity, I had to decide what to do. Was I going to become a Lyme patient and take months of damaging antibiotics, perhaps to no effect, and possibly triggering more autoimmune disease? And if I did pursue treatment, whom was I to trust, and how far would I go—would I take years of antibiotics without having a clear-cut positive test for the infection or knowing if my symptoms were caused by bacteria instead of my own immune system?

A FEW NIGHTS LATER, I was distracted from these questions by a reminder of exactly what Western medicine did well. On a warm October night, after Jim and I attended our friend Chris's sixtieth birthday party at a bar off Sixth Avenue, I went to bed feeling achy. I dreamed that I was walking down a long dark street and from a corner a shadowy figure in a trench coat leapt out and began stabbing me. Blood oozed through my hands as I clutched my side.

Covered in sweat, I woke. Our upstairs neighbor was awake in her bedroom, with a guest; I heard low voices. The stabbing was still there. I lurched from the bed, got a glass of water, took an Advil, and tried to go back to sleep. The pain, I suspected from experience, was from my endometriosis. Usually it passed within an hour. I told myself, *It's just pain,* and bit my hand to distract myself from it.

This time, though, the pain mounted instead of passing. Jim had been working late in the other room. I found him asleep on the couch, his laptop softly whirring on his chest. I woke him. Startled, he looked at me in confusion. "Get the car, please," I said. "You have to take me to the hospital."

The pain was intensely located in one place on my right lower abdomen—I visualized it as a dime-sized spot of radioactive light—but now it radiated outward. It was so severe I thought I couldn't remain in the box that was my body anymore—and yet I had to. I found myself thinking deliriously of the scene in *Dune* when the young Paul Atreides undergoes the gom jabbar test: he is asked by the religious leaders to put his hand in a box that inflicts painful nerve induction to identify if a person can use will to overcome animal instinct. Death is the consequence of the failure to overcome pain. If he removes his hand, he will be pricked by the poisoned gom jabbar. I, too, wanted to escape the pain, but the only way would be to die, I thought. Instead, I suddenly vomited.

As I waited for Jim to show up with the car, it occurred to me that the pain might mean I was dying, and I reflected, with strange calm, on how I would ask him to prepare. I wanted him to throw out the bad drafts of poems on my computer but salvage anything he thought worth keeping. The door opened, Jim rushed into the room, got me into the car, holding my hand at traffic lights. Every time the car hit a pothole I inhaled sharply.

When we got to the hospital at three a.m., the lobby was empty and cavernous, an abandoned temple. I was a topiary of nerves. As I got through the sliding glass doors my knees buckled. People in pastel scrubs materialized with a wheelchair and wound me through many bright halls and into an elevator, speaking softly, and then in a large cold room someone took my name, which I could barely remember, and before I knew it there was the pinch of a needle in my inner arm and morphine hitting my bloodstream. The pain diminished slightly. I stopped retching. A doctor came to examine me and pressed my abdomen so hard I screamed. Then he called the student over and said, "Press here," and I screamed again. "Could you stop doing that?" I snapped.

It turned out I had an endometrial cyst that had ruptured and now was bleeding throughout my pelvic cavity, and the doctors were considering emergency surgery if I lost too much blood. I was whisked through many exams and a sonogram and then to a bed, where they kept me hooked up to morphine, which had the effect of dissolving all my fear. As it kicked in, a hazy tranquility came with it. "I feel so safe," I kept telling the attending doctors and the residents coming in and out of the room.

The doctors monitored me. At first the internal bleeding did not stop. They started an IV to hydrate me and continue delivering morphine and even sent an acupressure specialist to my bed to help manage the pain through touch. Eventually, the bleeding slowed, and my blood pressure stabilized. This was Western medicine at its best. I needed the painkillers; I needed the monitoring. The doctors made me feel safe and comfortable, even if no one asked me any personal questions beyond my name.

Because emergency surgery is never as safe as a planned surgery, they discharged me with the plan to conduct surgery to remove the remnants of the cyst on Christmas Eve. My surgeon did it with great efficiency, and by evening I was home, exchanging gifts with friends by the glow of our Christmas tree, high on oxycodone, which made the entire episode seem like a strange dream, and me still in it, watching those I love fold their limbs below them as they pulled the shiny gold paper off boxes.

FOURTEEN

NADIR

In the dark and bitterly cold days of the winter of 2013, as I weighed contacting a Lyme doctor for a second opinion on my lab results, I believed I was dying. I would attempt to will myself to work for an hour only to find myself back in bed, asleep. For days on end, the bed was my landscape. It stretched around me like the plains. My mind was occupied with waiting until the pain and discomfort passed. I understood certain aspects of madness better, the nearly rote repetitions that come when meaning has faltered on the inside. Any outing—to teach my classes, mainly—meant days of recovery afterward. I got more blood work, more IV vitamin drips, and followed Dr. C's protocols. I took steroids in case they might help with hidden autoimmune issues. I only got sicker.

"Can't this be *over*?" I whispered to my computer screen.

One chilly night, I drove a few colleagues from Princeton back to Brooklyn after a department holiday party. I looked over at the man sitting next to me—a novelist I'd known for years—and realized I had no idea who he was. I knew I *knew* him, but who was he? It took an hour to recover the information that he was a friend and a colleague. At home, I asked Jim whether he had ever experienced anything like this. He shook his head.

I find it hard to write about the nadir that was that winter. In some ways this is the point: the annihilating absence of language, the impossibility of finding a story to tell about the blankness that confronted me day after day, the chasm between me and other humans. Even now, as intensely unbearable as those months were, what words do I have? "Fatigue" and "pain" hardly cut it; they are anti-dramatic, general, abstract. I don't have other words to use. There wasn't, after all, the stink of blood pooling on the floor; a mangled limb; the pallor of high fever. Instead, a grayness crept over me. The image I had was of a person slowly having her life force sucked out of her, like Pepito in Ludwig Bemelmans's *Madeline in London*, who becomes terribly homesick after he moves away from the twelve little girls and grows "thin" and then "thinner."

I caught myself wondering, again, if my symptoms were the manifestation solely of a depression so extreme it had utterly fooled me. But a low pilot flame of myself kept insisting, *I'm here, I want to get better.*

Some of Dr. C's protocols—the phosphatidylcholine IV drip—briefly made me feel better. But the overall arc was downward. And yet I still resisted the idea that I might have late-stage Lyme. It might strain credulity that a person who believes she is dying doesn't just try some antibiotics, especially after all the experimental treatments I had tried. But when I mind-tunnel back in time, I can briefly reinhabit how convinced I was that the autoimmune issues would only get worse if I took antibiotics—and how skeptical I was that I had Lyme disease. I knew a woman who, like me, had received indeterminate Lyme-disease tests; she pursued expensive and elaborate treatment and realized later that she had a systemic autoimmune condition characterized by pain and fatigue that had gone undetected by doctors.

I had long been haunted by the idea that something was wrong with me that *could* be fixed, that the answer was out there, right in front of us, but no one else was looking for it.

But I had not anticipated what should have been my biggest fear of all: that I would lose hope.

In *Darkness Visible: A Memoir of Madness,* William Styron writes about a journal he didn't want others to see. He always knew that if he "decided to get rid of the notebook that moment would necessarily coincide with my decision to put an end to myself." One morning that winter, as I woke early and sat on the couch, clicking through recipes I didn't have the energy to make, my mind hitched on the urgent need to delete my writing files. I had always told myself that before I approached the end of my life, I would delete the writing I didn't want anyone seeing.

Without quite noticing it, I had slid downward to a place where, as Styron put it, "all sense of hope had vanished, along with the idea of a futurity." My research into what could be making me feel so unwell had slowed to a standstill. An apprehension of death settled over me. I was not entirely surprised years later to find, rereading Styron's book, how similar were the experience of major depression and the inchoate suffering I underwent. In his case, in the afternoon he would "feel the horror, like some poisonous fogbank, roll in upon my mind, forcing me into bed. There I would lie for as long as six hours, stuporous and virtually paralyzed, gazing at the ceiling."

The difference was that my fog was caused by fatigue and pain, which of course were slowly allowing despair to crowd in. But this description— the poisonous fogbank!—evoked the miasma I was trapped in, the hours of stupor, the white couch cushion that had gradually turned gray from the contact with my jeans where I sat, day after day. Once it had been the case that by late morning the fog in my brain would clear, and I would have a few good hours in which I could work or read. This was no longer true. By eleven a.m., a fatigue of stunning density would wash upward through my body. I would head to bed, where I would sleep for three or four hours at a time, dreaming of forgetting to go to class or neglecting to show up at a reading I was scheduled to give.

That winter was extraordinarily cold, and in late January it was always dark. In the subway there was a massive billboard for a new TV show that read DID I REALLY DIE? *Indeed,* I thought. One morning, I sat on the couch drinking my tea. I looked out the window, and my vision swam; the dark, contorted limbs of the tree in our front yard morphed ominously into the body of a tortured and self-knotted being.

I thought about the mind-body problem, which philosophers call "the hard problem." What did consciousness mean? I was not myself, but if I was not myself, how did I *know* that? It was as if the old me, the authentic me, were inside, struggling to break free of the forces that had inhabited its body. The ghost within.

I was, perhaps, a ghost.

But the fact that I felt like a ghost instead of merely feeling numb gave me a speck of hope.

Ghosts haunt themselves into being.

ONE WEEK IN JANUARY 2014, after I'd gone to get an IV vitamin treatment, Jim and I had a fight. In my desperation to find relief, a name, help, I had been going to see every practitioner who had been recommended to me, and all these visits cost money I did not have. I had been to many top doctors who no longer took insurance, and now, many fees later, I was broke and stressed. My credit card balances were piling up. "You need to take on more freelance work," Jim said. I looked at him blankly.

"Do you really not understand?" I said. "It takes me weeks to write what would once have taken me a few days."

"It's just . . . you're doing all this crazy stuff and you're paying so much money for it," he said in frustration. "How do you have *any* idea if it's helping? Why are you choosing to spend your money so randomly? We can't afford this."

I went cold with rage, a white light behind my eyes. He was both right and deeply wrong.

"I wish the science were there to help me decide what to do," I said. "But it's not. And no one wants to get better more than I do. Can't you see that I am desperate? I feel like my life is over, and no one is helping me."

"But you can't just try anything," he said. "You don't know if it's safe to put these things in your body."

"You should leave," I said, unable to hear any more.

I was furious at Jim because I didn't have anyone else to be furious at. I was furious at being furious with him. I was furious because I felt I had no ally in this horrible experience. And yet wasn't sympathy what you were supposed to get when you were sick? Jim understood something was wrong. But the conversation was a stark reminder that even he could only grasp a bit of what I was going through, and that my actions looked irrational when in fact they were the product of despairing calculations.

Jim shrugged and walked to the other side of the apartment, where he busied himself fiddling with the television.

I burst into tears. I wanted to be analytical about what was happening to me. But I now felt so optionless I was willing to do things that seemed less and less likely to pan out.

I can't remember now what happened or how we reconciled, only that we did. But between us there was a growing fissure around the issue of my illness.

Later that night, when I talked to him about it, Jim said, "I don't think you know how hard it is to watch, and watch, and watch, and not be able to do anything—not be able to help." He paused. "It's a very odd position to be in, to care, to see that you *are* sick, and to be so completely unable to help."

. . .

I DID NOT INJECT BLEACH into my veins—per Donald Trump's infamous suggestion to coronavirus patients—but Jim was right that I was taking new kinds of risks. I wish I could skip this part of the story. An integrative doctor I'd seen had suggested I try ozone and ultraviolet light therapy, in which blood is withdrawn, exposed to ultraviolet light, infused with molecular oxygen, and then put back in the body. I'd recoiled then, but now, from my exhausted posture on the couch, I thought, *What do I have to lose?*

In this manner, I put myself in the hands of someone I would not have trusted had I been less vulnerable. Decisions like this are often portrayed as products of the patient's credulousness, her naïveté. But the reality is that many of us are people who, faced with no good choice, shrug our way into the hands of those we don't trust in search of help.

Dr. G's office was in a sleek skyscraper with an imposing front desk but no detectable security. The walls of the office were painted a pastel shade that was more nauseating than cheerful. A nurse whisked me into his office. "Here you go," she said timorously, as the doctor jumped up from behind an enormous computer on his desk.

Dr. G—and he did have an MD, somehow—had curls that sprang wildly from his head. Even as I sat down, he was pulling a picture out of his desk drawer. "You see these bruises?" he said, handing me the photo. "They appeared after I treated her."

I was looking at a Polaroid of a young woman with Slavic features who appeared to be in her early twenties. She was brunette, thin, with an air of despair. A spray of bruises glowed on her arm.

"These diseases are caused by hidden trauma," Dr. G said, eagerly. "Her husband was beating her and she wasn't telling anyone. When I gave her the ozone, bruises appeared all over her body. She told me what was going on, and now she's better."

The woman looked barely old enough to vote. The fact that he had shown me her picture—the fact that he kept it in his desk—made me uncomfortable. Shifting backward in my chair, I winced. I was wearing a neck brace for the partially ruptured disc in my cervical spine, which I had reinjured a few days earlier. He looked me up and down and cried, "You've got degenerate neck disease!"

"Do you mean 'degenerative'?" I asked.

"Chronic degenerative disease of the sort you've got," he continued, "is caused by tooth decay!" He spoke as if he were singing in a musical: three out of four of his sentences were exclamatory. "Have you ever had a root canal?"

I nodded.

"Root canals harbor vicious bacteria! A surprising number of people who have had dental work have heart disease. It's because the low-level infection strains the body. But"—he leaned close—"I know how to help you. Ozone!"

He gazed at me, waiting for a response. When I gave none—frozen in horror—he grew stern. "And! You must have all your teeth with root canals pulled and replaced."

"Really?"

"Oh yes," he assured me. "Here," he said, leaning toward his computer screen, "let me show you. A man named Weston Price discovered that most illness is caused by the disgusting accumulation of bacteria that linger in root canals . . ."

"I'm pretty sure that subsequent research has discredited that theory," I interrupted. "They've examined root canals done with modern methods and haven't found horrific amounts of pathogenic bacteria growing in the canals. Haven't they?"

Dr. G turned red, one finger on the screen beside Weston Price's face.

"Well," he said, "I've had mine done and I feel great. My wife won't do them, even though I tell her to; she has all kinds of problems."

Whatever the science ultimately shows about ozone and ultraviolet irradiation therapy, what distresses me now about the memory is that I went along with the treatment even though I didn't trust Dr. G. He was the first doctor I met from the integrative tradition who seemed like an outright quack. For one thing, he was strangely insistent that I believe in him. I could feel his desire to convince me as intensely as my doctors must have felt my own desire to convert them to my cause. (Suddenly I experienced a surge of sympathy for them.) He told me that he had pioneered this treatment. He said that it was used in Germany, with full support of the national health care system. The implication was that American doctors were too blinkered or beholden to pharmaceutical companies to embrace it. Because ozone and UV aren't drugs, he said, there's no Big Pharma to back the studies of its efficacy. This seems plausible. But Germany's insurance system doesn't reimburse patients for ozone therapy either.

Dr. G and I headed to the treatment room. In this procedure, one hundred cubic centimeters—about a half cup—of blood is drawn out of you and irradiated with ultraviolet light, which supposedly kills bacteria and viruses that lead to infections, and strengthens the immune system. UV therapy is often combined with another procedure, known as "oxidative therapy," in which ozone or hydrogen peroxide is infused in the blood. The powerful "oxidants," which are molecules used in energy production, allegedly can help the white blood cells fight off infections. They also gently stress your body, said Dr. G, leading it to produce more antioxidants. In this procedure, UV and ozone are used together.

Like many alternative treatments, UV and ozone therapy is metaphorically appealing: after seeing many professionals, trying many drugs, having surgeries, it is wonderful to think that perhaps all you need is a concentrated dose of sunlight and fresh oxygen infused in your veins. And I knew that there were some forms of UV therapy—directed at the skin, say—that are beneficial for certain diseases.

In a room so small it felt like a closet, Dr. G made me drink some apple juice. Then he hooked me up to an IV that ran tubes into a machine that looked like a vintage IBM Selectric. It was tan and ugly, a large, flat rectangle, with tubes crisscrossing through it. He lifted the tubing and wound it through the machine, then pricked a vein in my elbow with a needle. Soon my blood flushed through the tubes.

"I turn on the UV light," he said, "then I inject oxygen, so you get your blood cleaned by the UV and oxygenated, to help your body fight the viruses you have."

The machine whirred peculiarly, antiquatedly. As my blood drained out of me, it turned a deep red after the UV and oxygen hit it and pooled in a bag.

"Ooh, your blood is really dark," he said. "That suggests you're sick."

With a cold hand, he took my arm, inspected my fingers, and told me that my nails were pale.

"Do your feet itch? You know, athlete's foot, that kind of thing?"

I shook my head, doing my best to ignore him. The machine clicked.

"Hmm, OK," he said. "Now we run the blood back in." Flicking a switch, he wiggled the IV needle in my vein. The bright blood ran back down the tubes. My blood was frothy with ozone; I started to feel sick as it ran back into me.

He shook the bag of blood. "This will help strip the viruses out," he said.

"Has this ever gone through peer review?" I asked.

"Are you feeling faint?" he responded. He peered at my face. I did feel queasy. My brain had filled with scraggly gray lines. "Your skin is shiny! Drink this. You're having a reaction." I closed my eyes and waved the apple juice away.

Outside the room an ambulance wailed. The machine *beep-beep-beeped* beside me. I heard a plane's engine drone past. I opened my eyes.

Another patient wheeled by in the hall—heavyset, in his fifties, IV in his arm—and winked at me.

"A vitamin drip!" he cried.

For twenty-four hours after Dr. G's treatment I felt a little worse, as I nearly always did after any kind of intervention. But then I felt better. For about three weeks my energy returned, frisking through the unused corners of my mind. My brain cleared. But I was left with the sour, dismaying sense that I had allowed a person I didn't trust to do something to me because I was out of options. Later, a nurse at another integrative practice would tell me that ozone treatment was something she would never try because she felt it carried too many risks.

By late January 2014, my headaches, brain fog, and joint pain had gotten worse, and tiny bruises had bloomed all over my legs and arms. I fainted several times. A black ocean, it seemed, kept crashing over me, so that I couldn't catch my breath. I could no more touch the old delights of my life than a firefly could touch the world beyond the jar in which it had been caught. I was only thirty-seven.

I began to feel terrified of staying alive like this. What if I could get my health back but only at the cost of having no sense of pleasure or interest in anything? Before I got sick, my work made my life meaningful. I wanted to be what Jenny Offill describes, in her novel *Dept. of Speculation*, as an "art monster": a woman who gives herself over to her art with an obsessiveness that forsakes the more conventional realities of a woman's life. When I got sick, my hunger for art remained intact, but my brain would not cooperate in helping me make and consume it.

Until recently, as sick as I was feeling, poems and art still had their shine. But that February, poems that used to make my limbic system shiver felt almost like news of a world I couldn't join. One morning I reread John Ashbery's "A Blessing in Disguise," a poem that had always stirred me with its evocation of the way desire makes us alive to the world:

> . . . I, in my soul, am alive too.
> I feel I must sing and dance, to tell
> Of this in a way, that knowing you may be drawn to me.
>
> And I sing amid despair and isolation
> Of the chance to know you, to sing of me
> Which are you. You see,
> You hold me up to the light in a way
>
> I should never have expected, or suspected, perhaps
> Because you always tell me I am you,
> And right. . . .

But the words felt remote.

The next day, I began deleting my writing files. I went online to my financial accounts and checked that I had labeled beneficiaries for each. I sat with my computer and went through file by file, deleting spare files, then went to the cabinet where my journals were kept. I hesitated, then piled them on a corner of the office shelving to bring out later with the garbage. It is hard to write about this time, but it would also be false to suggest that my illness had not at this point—two and half years into feeling that I had the flu every single day—led to despair about whether I could go on, without at least the prospect of my suffering being seen. For those weeks, I felt the depression at one's state that many chronically ill people confront at some point in their illness. (Research suggests that roughly one third of people with a serious medical condition experience symptoms of depression.) In no way do I think, or want to suggest, that depression was the *root* cause of my symptoms or my illness. Rather, in retrospect it is painfully clear that the *invisibility* of my illness was one of the most challenging parts of my suffering, wearing my resilience down over time. I have always been a social person who thrives on deep connection with others. Like many type-A personalities, I was willing to work extremely hard, and accommodate myself to a great deal of pain, if a doctor just told me what to do and expect, or if I knew that my illness was being meaningfully researched. But the near total absence of recognition of how sick I was confounded me: it rendered my suffering meaningless.

Recently I found a scrap of a story I started writing on my iPhone during this time. It opens, "When I woke it was clear they had been erasing my memories again. Their faces loomed forward and receded. I couldn't tell what their eyes said." Those sentences say a great deal about how disconnected I had grown from the hope that had so far propelled me to search for answers. It is easy to see now that the image of an anonymous "they" erasing my memories was a metaphor for my sense of being invisible, and the absence of meaning that came with it. A person without memory is a person without meaning.

Only a few friends realized at the time how much physical suffering I was undergoing. We are bad at recognizing the suffering of others unless we are given clear-cut clues and evidence. And so invisible illnesses often go unacknowledged, while less serious conditions get attention.

Years later, pregnant with my first son, I had a terrible allergic reaction to a medication I was taking, and my skin became scaly and inflamed, from my face to my feet. Everyone who saw me said, "That looks miserable," and doctors rushed to relieve my symptoms.

"You must be very uncomfortable," one said.

"Poor thing," volunteered another.

But this rash, as terrible as it was, was nothing compared to what I had felt when I was at my most ill. The difference was that none of these symptoms could be seen. The illness was severe but invisible. And that invisibility made all the difference—it made *me* invisible, which itself almost killed me.

. . .

ONE MARCH DAY I met up with my friend Katie, who had a new baby. She was waiting for me in the coffee shop on a narrow wooden pew, reclaimed from a local church that had been turned into condominiums, as an icy snow stung the ground outside. The baby was sleeping in his stroller beside her, swaddled and peaceful in a way few adults ever seem to be. We sat and talked about her new baby, the novel she was writing, an acquaintance in the midst of a divorce. As customers gathered, the windows steamed up and made the room cozy and warm, the yellow light a cocoon. Her baby woke unexpectedly, and she picked him up and lifted him to her with a smile that pierced me. I wasn't missing only life's bacchanalian pleasures—the pleasure of tart raspberries and custard, the self-forgetfulness of a muscle-burning workout, the energetic sense of hurtling out the door, excited about a meeting—but its metaphysical ones. I had no children, and I wanted to be a mother. I once had ambition and yearned to write; now I only wanted the pain and fog to lift. I was, in some profound sense, interrupted and out of time, and it was this—the gray-wool hours through which I moved, the loss of a life as a mother, the loss of meaningful work—that pained me more than anything.

Katie laughed, jerking me out of my thoughts. The baby was smiling and cooing at her, his hair flicked softly up and to the side, his skin untarnished.

I was flooded with a hunger for life that I had not experienced in weeks. *I really want to get better,* I thought. *No, not "better." I want to have the will to keep living with this illness.*

A sense of hope rushed in. I knew then that I needed to learn more about the complex reality of Lyme disease and tackle the near-impossible task of sorting out what was understood and what was not. At the recommendation of a science-writer friend, I finally made an appointment to go to upstate New York to see Richard Horowitz, a Lyme specialist, who is an internist with a focus on the disease.

I did not yet know that simply by exploring whether untreated Lyme disease could be the cause of my illness, I risked being labeled one of the "Lyme loonies"—patients who believed that a long-ago bite from a tick was the cause of their years of suffering. They had been called that in a 2007 email sent by the program officer overseeing Lyme grants at the National Institutes of Health. The now-infamous phrase betrayed just how fiercely contested the disease is—"one of the biggest controversies that medicine has seen," as John Aucott, a physician and the director of the Johns Hopkins Lyme Disease Research Center, later described it to me. And I was walking right into the middle of it.

FIFTEEN

LYME DISEASE

I rode the train to my appointment with Dr. Horowitz, traveling alongside the deep blue Hudson River. The office, when I arrived after a short taxi ride from Poughkeepsie, was quieter than I expected. A teenage girl in a wheelchair and her mother sat near me. Behind the receptionist, stickers with bitter jokes about Lyme disease were plastered on the file cabinets. The tiles of the linoleum floor were arranged in mandalas.

Horowitz, who goes by "Dr. H" with many of his patients, is a practicing Buddhist, with bright-blue eyes and an air of brimming eagerness. He recently served as a member of the Tick-Borne Disease Working Group convened by the Department of Health and Human Services, which in 2018 issued a report to Congress outlining problems with the diagnosis and treatment of Lyme patients.

When I saw him, I told him that I wasn't sure I had Lyme disease. I had brought along a stack of lab results nearly half a foot tall—a paper trail that would scare off many doctors. As we sat there, I felt foolish. Surely this was silly and I did not really have Lyme. But Horowitz perused every page of my labs, asking questions and making notes. Finally, almost an hour after we began, he sighed and looked up.

"Based on your labs, your symptoms, and your various results over the years, I highly suspect you have Lyme," he said. "See these?" He bent over a set of results from a lab at Stony Brook. "These bands are specific for Lyme."

"But what about the fact that the results seemed to be mixed?" I asked.

He sighed again. "Let me explain something about the tests."

Heading to Dr. H's office that day, I hadn't known what I was in for. Imperfect diagnostics lie at the core of the whole debate over Lyme disease. Standard Lyme tests—structured in two tiers, to minimize false positives—can neither reliably identify an infection early on nor determine whether an infection has been eradicated. This is because no test can dependably identify whether a person has the spirochete that causes Lyme disease in their blood. Instead, the tests look for the antibodies (those small proteins our bodies create to fight infection) produced in response to the bacteria. But antibody production takes time, and this means that early detection can be problematic. (Even someone who has a bull's-eye rash, for instance, can test negative.) And once produced, antibodies can last for years, which makes it difficult to see whether an infection is resolved, or even whether a new one has occurred. Furthermore, antibodies to autoimmune and viral diseases can resemble the ones the body makes in response to Lyme.

For a thorough interpretive reading, some doctors will send blood to several different labs, which can deliver results that do not always agree with one another. The CDC recommends that only a specific pattern of antibodies, agreed on by experts in 1994, be considered indicative of a positive test. But it also suggests that when necessary, doctors should use their judgment to make a clinical diagnosis, based on symptoms and likelihood of exposure, along with the lab tests.

In my case, I had two tests that showed I was positive for an array of antibodies particular to Lyme disease, but I lacked the short-term anti-bodies that usually signal that you have been infected.

In Horowitz's waiting room, I had filled out an elaborate question-naire designed to differentiate Lyme patients from a pool of patients with other illnesses. (It has been empirically validated as a screening tool.) Now Dr. H did a physical exam and ordered a range of tests to rule out further thyroid problems, diabetes, and other possible causes of my symptoms. He mentioned that some people with persistent Lyme symptoms may have what is a called a "co-infection": a second or even third infection transmitted by the tick, such as bartonella, to take just one example. Because I had night sweats and the sensation that I couldn't get enough air into my lungs (a symptom known as "air hunger") he suggested that I might have a co-infection of babesia, a malaria-like parasite also transmitted by ticks. Curious, I told him that I had always thought of Lyme as a primarily arthritic disease, whereas I had many neurological and cognitive symptoms. He explained that the Lyme bac-terium is now known to come in different strains, which are thought to produce different kinds of diseases.

Dr. H also talked about the fact that the people who got sickest from Lyme may also have a host of overlapping issues, such as food sensitivi-ties and gut dysbiosis, autoimmune disease, mold exposure, genetic is-sues, thyroid disease, and problems of the nervous system, such as dysautonomia.

"The funny thing is, I think you're actually a very strong and healthy person, and that's why you did OK for so long," he continued. "Now your body needs help."

Dr. H prescribed a month of doxycycline and warned me about something I had also read about online. When I began the antibiotic, I might at first feel worse: as the bacteria die, they release toxins that create what's known as a "Jarisch-Herxheimer reaction"—a flu-like response that Lyme patients commonly refer to as "herxing." But over time, he said, I should feel better. If not, we were on the wrong track.

Over dinner that night I told Jim that despite what Horowitz had urged, I still wasn't sure I wanted to take the antibiotics. I hadn't had a cut-and-dried positive test for Lyme, and I knew how damaging antibiotics are to the microbiome. "What do you have to lose?" he asked in disbelief. "You're sick, you're suffering, and you've tried everything else."

Today, I share Jim's disbelief. Looking back now, I can see that to him my reluctance must have seemed bizarre: I had tried so many outlandish remedies and been so willing to chase down any possibility, however slim. Now, when I suddenly had a lead, why would I refuse to try antibiotics—a basic component of modern medicine, a drug I'd taken many times before? For one thing, I had absorbed the notion that unnecessary antibiotic use in my childhood had probably helped contribute to my autoimmune disease. Then, too, I see now, I had lost hope. To embark on a new path was almost beyond me.

"Just try it," Jim said, urgently. "The antibiotics can't possibly make you much worse than you are right now." And so I got a glass of water to take the first pill.

LYME DISEASE WAS DISCOVERED IN Connecticut in the mid-1970s. Today, it is a major, and growing, health threat whose reach extends well beyond its initial East Coast locus. Reported cases increased almost fivefold from 1992 to 2017, and the Centers for Disease Control and Prevention estimates that annual incidence has risen to more than three hundred thousand. "There is little question that Lyme is on the rise," Richard Ostfeld, a disease ecologist at the Cary Institute of Ecosystem Studies, told me. The CDC has named babesia, the co-infection Horowitz thought I might have, a significant concern for the national blood supply. A time-lapse epidemiological map I saw at a conference at Massachusetts General Hospital showed a steady spread of red from 1976, from Long Island, the Connecticut shoreline, and Martha's Vineyard, westward and northward and southward, until it had saturated the coast of the Northeast a disconcertingly bloody crimson. Lyme disease and other tick-borne illnesses are now prevalent in Northern California, Minnesota, Wisconsin, and southern states like Virginia. Cases of Lyme disease have now been found in every state, and in many parts of Europe. Step into parks not just in coastal Maine, but even in Paris, and you'll see ominous signs warning of the presence of the ticks that carry Lyme disease. In the summer in the eastern United States, many parents I know cover their children from head to toe—never mind the heat—for a hike in the woods or a jaunt to a grassy playground.

By now, just about everyone knows someone who's been diagnosed with Lyme disease, and most of us know to look for the telltale rash (although they are often described as a bull's-eye, many Lyme rashes are solid-colored lesions) and to ask for a prompt dose of antibiotics. For most of those who are swiftly diagnosed and treated, that will be the end of the story. But many Americans have also heard secondhand reports of people who did not get well after their course of antibiotics, or of cases in which no rash appeared and a diagnosis came late, after much damage had been wrought. Many others, upon discovering an attached deer tick, have encountered doctors who balk at prescribing anything to treat a possible Lyme infection, wary of overdiagnosis and overuse of antibiotics.

The alarm and confusion surrounding such a long-standing public health issue is extraordinary. The consequences cannot be overestimated, now that Lyme disease has become—the pandemic aside—an almost "unparalleled threat to regular American life," as Bennett Nemser, a former Columbia University epidemiologist who manages the Cohen Lyme and Tickborne Disease Initiative at the Steven & Alexandra Cohen Foundation, characterized it to me. "Really anyone—regardless of age, gender, political interest, affluence—can touch a piece of grass and get a tick on them."

Even as changes in the climate and in land use are contributing to a dramatic rise in Lyme and other tick-borne diseases, the American medical establishment remains entrenched in a struggle over who can be said to have Lyme disease and whether it can become chronic—and if so, why. The standoff has impeded research that could clarify how a wily bacterium, and the co-infections that can come with it, can affect human bodies. After forty years in the public health spotlight, Lyme disease still eludes reliable testing, still cannot be prevented by a vaccine (Valneva and Pfizer are at work on one they hope will be in use by 2025), and still pits patients against doctors and researchers against one another. When I got my inconclusive diagnosis, I knew better than to dream of a quick cure. But I had no idea how extreme the roller coaster of uncertainty would be.

LYME DISEASE CAME INTO public view when an epidemic of what appeared to be rheumatoid arthritis began afflicting children in Lyme, Connecticut. A young rheumatologist at Yale named Allen Steere, who went on to conduct research at Massachusetts General Hospital in Boston, studied the children. In 1976, he named the mysterious illness after its locale and described its main symptoms more fully: a bull's-eye rash, fevers and aches, Bell's palsy (partial paralysis of the face) and other neurological issues, and rheumatological manifestations such as swelling of the knees. After much study, Steere realized that the black-legged ticks that live on mice and deer (among other mammals) might be harboring a pathogen responsible for the outbreak. In 1981, the medical entomologist Willy Burgdorfer finally identified the bacterium that causes Lyme, and it was named after him: *Borrelia burgdorferi*.

B. burgdorferi is a corkscrew-shaped bacterium (called a spirochete) that can burrow deep into its host's tissue, causing damage as it goes and, in laboratory conditions at least, transforming as needed from corkscrew to cyst-like blob to slimy biofilm forms. Because of this ability, researchers describe it as an "immune evader." Once it hits the human bloodstream, it changes its outer surface to elude an immune response and then quickly moves from the blood into tissue, which poses problems for early detection. (Hard to find in the bloodstream and other body fluids, the *B. burgdorferi* spirochete is difficult to culture, which is how bacterial infections are definitively diagnosed.) If it goes untreated, *B. burgdorferi* can make its way into fluid in the joints, into the spinal cord, and even into the brain and the heart, where it can cause the sometimes-deadly Lyme carditis.

By the mid-1990s, a mainstream consensus emerged that Lyme disease was relatively easy to diagnose, thanks to the telltale rash and flu-like symptoms, as well as to treat. Infectious diseases are the kind of clear-cut illness that our medical system generally excels at handling. Evidence indicated that the prescribed treatment protocol—a few weeks of oral antibiotics, typically doxycycline—would take care of most cases that were caught early, while late-stage cases of Lyme disease (instances when the infection had gone untreated and the bacteria had disseminated through the body) might require intravenous antibiotics for up to a month. That assessment, made by the Infectious Diseases Society of America (IDSA), formed the basis of the IDSA's treatment guidelines from 2006 until recently. In late June 2019, a revised draft called for, among other things, a shorter course—ten days—of doxycycline for patients with early Lyme.

But the picture on the ground looked far murkier. A significant percentage of people who had Lyme symptoms and later tested positive for the disease had never gotten the rash. Others had many characteristic symptoms but tested negative for the infection, yet entered treatment anyway. And a portion of patients who had been promptly and conclusively diagnosed with Lyme disease and treated with the standard course of doxycycline never got well. When people from each of these groups failed to recover fully, they began referring to their condition as "chronic Lyme disease," believing in some cases that bacteria were still lurking deep in their bodies.

Frustrated with the medical system's seeming inability to help them, patients emerged as an activist force, arguing that Lyme disease was harder to cure in some people than the establishment acknowledged.

Family physicians in Lyme-endemic areas, confronted with patients who remained ill, tried out other treatment protocols, including long-term oral and intravenous antibiotics, sometimes administered for months or years. They also started testing assiduously for tick-borne co-infections, which were appearing in some of the sickest patients. Many of these doctors rotated drugs in the hope of finding a more effective regimen. Some patients responded well. Others did not. In 1999, these doctors banded together to form the International Lyme and Associated Diseases Society (ILADS). Highlighting the problems with Lyme-disease tests and citing early evidence that bacteria could persist in animals and humans with Lyme disease even after they had been treated, ILADS proposed an alternative standard of care that defines the illness more broadly, allows for more extensive treatment, and recognizes that Lyme infections can leave people sick for years.

But some prominent Lyme-disease scientists were skeptical that the infection could persist after treatment—that the bacterium could remain in the body. They argued that many chronic-Lyme-disease patients were being treated for an infection they no longer had, while others had never had Lyme disease in the first place but had appropriated the diagnosis for symptoms that could easily have other causes. Chronic Lyme disease, in the Infectious Diseases Society of America's view, was a pseudoscientific diagnosis—an ideology rather than a biological reality, unsupported by medical evidence. Under the sway of that ideology, the IDSA contended, credulous patients were needlessly being treated with dangerous IV antibiotics by irresponsible physicians. (The IDSA case got a boost when a Lyme patient in her thirties died from an IV-related infection.) To prove that the bacterium was not causing the ongoing symptoms patients were reporting, the IDSA cited a handful of studies indicating that long-term antibiotic treatment of patients with such symptoms was no more effective than a placebo.

Instead of devoting compassion and energy to patients with persistent symptoms, many doctors focused on discrediting their testimony. The IDSA highlighted statistics suggesting that the commonly cited chronic Lyme symptoms—ongoing fatigue, brain fog, joint pain—occurred no more frequently in Lyme patients than in the general population. In the press, experts in the IDSA camp implied that patients who believed they had been sick with Lyme disease for years were deluded or mentally ill.

The antagonism was "fierce and alienating for the patients," Brian Fallon, the director of the Lyme and Tick-Borne Diseases Research Center at Columbia University Irving Medical Center, told me. Hostilities continued to intensify, not just between patients and experts but between community doctors and academic doctors. In 2006, the IDSA guidelines for patients and physicians included the warning that "in many patients, posttreatment symptoms appear to be more related to the aches and pains of daily living rather than to either Lyme disease or a tick-borne co-infection."

This message rang hollow for many. "Researchers were saying, 'Your symptoms have nothing to do with Lyme. You have chronic fatigue syndrome, or fibromyalgia, or depression,'" Fallon told me. "And that didn't make sense to these patients, who were well until they got Lyme, and then were sick."

The establishment's antagonism also helped to slow research into persistent symptoms, failing a generation of patients.

THE MORNING AFTER SEEING HOROWITZ, I took another dose of the doxycycline, along with Plaquenil, which is thought to help the antibiotics penetrate cells better. I took the third dose that night with dinner. I went to bed and woke up feeling like hell. My throat was sore and my head was foggy. My neck was a fiery rebar. I was extremely nauseated.

Two days later, we went out to get lunch. I was still groggy and unwell. It was a heavy, gray day, with low clouds. Returning home, I felt rain all over my bare arms. I told Jim we should hurry.

"Why?" he said.

"It's raining!"

"It's not raining," he said. "It's just cloudy." I raised my hands to show him the raindrops. A dozen pips of cold popped along my arm. But there was no rain. As we walked home, cold drops rushed all over my body, my skin crawling as if a strange, violent water were cleansing it.

Several days later, though, I felt excited about flying to a conference in Chicago rather than exhausted by the prospect. For three more weeks, I took the drugs and supplements Dr. H had prescribed. The doxycycline made me allergic to the sun. One cloudy late-spring morning, holding a coffee cup, I took a walk with Katie but had forgotten to put sunblock on my right hand. By the time I got home, my hand felt tender. Over the next few days a second-degree burn developed, blistering into an open wound.

After a month of antibiotic treatment, I took the train back up to Dr. H's office. On his questionnaire, I rated my symptoms as less severe than I had a month earlier, but my total score still fell in the high range. Dr. H changed the antibiotic protocol, and added Mepron, an antimalarial drug. He was concerned about my continued night sweats and air hunger.

Because I was still having bouts of dizziness, he decided to test me for a condition called "POTS," or "postural orthostatic tachycardia syndrome," which many of his patients suffered from. POTS is a subtype of dysautonomia. ("Dysautonomia," as mentioned earlier, is itself an umbrella term for a host of different conditions, many of whose causes have yet to be fully pinned down.) In common manifestations of POTS, a patient's autonomic nervous system has trouble regulating the heart's response to exertion, changes in posture, or variations in temperature, sending the body into an inappropriate fight-or-flight response. Some patients' systems have trouble adjusting blood pressure or constricting blood vessels to send blood to the brain. Blood can pool in the legs and peripheries of the body. The heart might compensate by increasing its rate, while the body releases surges of adrenaline in a fruitless attempt to correct the problem. As a result, patients can experience some blend of fatigue, headaches, digestive problems, heart palpitations, and cognitive issues such as brain fog. (POTS has become better known of late because COVID-19 appears to trigger it, or a condition closely resembling it, in a significant number of patients.)

Given my repeated bouts of fainting, Dr. H wanted to evaluate me for POTS using an active stand test, where he would measure my heart rate and my blood pressure at regular intervals as I stood, after first establishing a baseline heart rate while I was sitting. If my heart rate kept increasing over time—specifically, if it climbed more than thirty beats per minute—while my blood pressure remained stable, it could mean I had POTS and that, among other things, my nervous system was not successfully driving blood to my head. It could explain some of my fatigue and dizziness.

A nurse slipped the blood pressure cuff on my arm as I sat on the exam table and told me to relax; I was clenching my fists. My resting heart rate was 63 and my blood pressure was 90/60. I stood, and she took my vitals again and told me to wait. She kept measuring as the minutes passed. Increasingly uncomfortable, I started to shift my weight. "Don't move," she cautioned. At ten minutes my heart rate was at 94 and my blood pressure remained the same. Dr. H came back in the room and looked at the results and suggested that I likely had POTS. I was advised to drink more water, eat more salt, and wear compression stockings—all of which help by creating more blood supply and preventing blood from pooling. POTS, he explained, usually wasn't curable, but these measures might help alleviate my symptoms and bring significantly better quality of life. "Let's see how you do before we consider medication."

I left Dr. H's office dazed: for years, I'd had no answers for so many of my symptoms and now, suddenly, I had many explanations—as well as validation. A number of things really *were* going wrong in different systems. I hadn't been imagining it. "You must be shaken," a friend said that night when I told her what the doctor had found. And I was—but it was also a relief just to know, to have a name for what was wrong.

At the same time, I had come to understand that there would not be *one* explanation, *one* label, *one* diagnosis for what was happening to me—I knew enough to know that living in uncertainty was my lot. The years of being ill had taught me that each diagnosis—Hashimoto's, endometriosis, Lyme, POTS, and later Ehlers-Danlos syndrome—came with its own separate set of symptoms. If diagnosis now hardly felt like the end point of my quest, it was nonetheless an important piece, and I was comforted to have an explanation for what had been a mysterious set of seemingly unrelated problems.

Later, a cardiologist at Mount Sinai, Amy Kontorovich, evaluated me for POTS after I had fainted in a hotel room and hit my head on a bathtub, receiving a serious concussion. She came up with even more striking findings; during an active stand test, my heart rate rose more than forty beats per minute. "You definitely have POTS," she said. "That explains the dizziness and the fainting. I suspect the POTS is playing a significant role in producing your symptoms," she said kindly, indicating that she was surprised it had taken me so long to get a formal diagnosis for something that was, after all, measurable. Kontorovich also diagnosed me with the genetic condition hypermobile Ehlers-Danlos syndrome, and told me that due to their impaired connective tissue, people with EDS often had POTS, fatigue, and chronic pain—it could be an explanation for my stubborn remaining symptoms.

. . .

WHEN I STARTED TAKING the new antibiotics, in June 2014, along with the Mepron and the salt for the POTS, I was nearly as sick as I had ever been. I flew to Paris to teach at NYU's summer writing program. Within two days of arriving, I could barely walk down the street. Violent electric shocks lacerated my skin, and patches of burning pain and numbness spread up my neck. I shook and shivered. The reaction lasted five days, during which panic mixed with the pain. How was I to know whether this was herxing—a positive reaction to the drugs as they killed bacteria and parasites—or a manifestation of the disease itself? Or if weeks of antibiotics and antimalarials were themselves causing problems for me?

"I know you think you're doing the right thing," a concerned colleague said, "but aren't you just making yourself sicker?"

On the sixth day, I was sitting on the couch in my rented apartment and the shocks were so violent, racing across my forearms and thighs and calves, that when I looked up at the tall open windows, the sun streaming through them, it occurred to me that I could jump out of them and find relief.

The next morning, I woke up to the same bright sun, feeling better than I had in ages. Stunned by my energy, I went out for a run. I wasn't exactly racing down the sidewalk, but forty minutes later, for the first time in years, I had run three miles. As the weeks passed, I felt better and better. My drenching night sweats vanished. The air hunger was gone. I had loads of energy.

BY THE TIME I STARTED my treatment, the fact that Lyme disease causes ongoing symptoms in some patients could no longer be viewed as the product of their imaginations. (Indeed, by now, in the era of COVID, the idea that an infection might leave some people sick for months no longer seems so strange.) A well-designed longitudinal study by John Aucott at Johns Hopkins showed the presence of persistent brain fog, joint pain, and related issues in approximately 10 percent of even an ideally treated population—patients who got the Lyme rash and took the recommended antibiotics. Other studies found these symptoms in up to 20 percent of patients. The condition, christened "post-treatment Lyme disease syndrome," or PTLDS, is now recognized by the CDC. Even so, the condition is hotly contested, and some high-level people in the field—as well as the Infectious Diseases Society of America itself—still refuse to recognize it as an official diagnosis. (After much reporting on this subject, I still don't fully understand why. It seems clear that PTLDS—whatever its cause—is real.) Perhaps most important, crucial questions about the cause of ongoing symptoms remain unanswered, due in part to the decades-long standoff over whether and how the disease can become chronic. As Sue Visser, the CDC's associate director for policy in the Division of Vector-Borne Diseases, acknowledges, "Many are very rightfully frustrated that it's been decades and we still don't have answers for some patients."

For decades there has been little federal funding to study Lyme disease. Recently, though, a host of new studies sponsored by private foundations, including the Steven & Alexandra Cohen Foundation, the Global Lyme Alliance, and the Bay Area Lyme Foundation, has freshly tackled a number of those questions: Why do Lyme symptoms persist in only some patients? What don't we know about the behavior of the *B. burgdorferi* bacterium that might help explain the variation in patients' responses to it?

It turns out that PTLDS (or chronic Lyme disease) brings us back to that old soil-and-seed model. Though the ongoing illness is triggered by a clear-cut infection, *B. burgdorferi* seems to be a bacterium that makes some people much sicker than others, for reasons scientists do not fully understand. It is not like other clear-cut infectious illness: the familiar model of "get exposed to the germ; catch a disease; treat it with a drug" does not apply. Rather, it may be that tick-borne illnesses—much as COVID-19 now seems to—trigger a vastly different array of immune responses in people.

In a conversation I had with him, Bennett Nemser of the Cohen Foundation laid out some of the hypotheses that are currently being explored. The complexity is daunting. A patient with ongoing symptoms may still have a Lyme infection and/or a lingering infection from some other tick-borne disease that was never diagnosed. Or the original infection might have caused systemic damage, leaving the patient with recurring symptoms such as nerve pain and chronic inflammation. Or the Lyme infection might have triggered an autoimmune response. Or, finally, the patient might be suffering from some combination of all three, complicated by triggers that researchers have not yet identified.

One way or another, new research suggests, an intricate interplay of the infection and the immune system is at work in patients who do not get better, just as it now seems to be at work in long COVID. The immune response to the Lyme infection is "highly variable," John Aucott told me. For example, some research has suggested that ongoing symptoms are a result of an overactive immune response triggered by Lyme disease. Recently, though, a study coauthored by Aucott with scientists at Stanford found that in patients who developed PTLDS, the Lyme bacterium had inhibited the immune response (making it more likely it could persist). In this sense, the researchers working on Lyme disease are at the forefront, too, of fresh insights into how an infection— or the debilitating consequences of successive infections—can activate chronic inflammatory diseases, sometimes destabilizing the nervous system and triggering dysautonomia.

In the meantime, accumulating evidence suggests that in many mammals Lyme bacteria can persist after treatment with antibiotics. In 2012, a team led by the microbiologist Monica Embers of the Tulane National Primate Research Center found intact *B. burgdorferi* lingering for months in rhesus macaques after treatment. Embers also reported that the macaques had varying immune responses to the infection, possibly explaining why active bacteria remained in some of the animals: their immune systems weren't sufficiently dispatching the pathogen. The study drew criticism from figures in the IDSA establishment, because it failed to prove that the bacteria remained biologically active. But Embers and her team have managed to culture *B. burgdorferi* in mice who had been treated with a course of doxycycline, showing that the bacterium can remain viable in animals after treatment.

Then, in May of 2021, Embers and Brian Fallon published a startling autopsy study in *Frontiers in Medicine*, reporting that they had found intact *Borrelia* spirochetes in the brain and central nervous system of a sixty-nine-year-old woman who had suffered from severe neuro-cognitive issues before her death. The woman had been diagnosed with Lyme disease fifteen years earlier and treated aggressively with antibiotics, which, according to the IDSA, should have wiped out the bacteria. The autopsy suggested that had not happened.

But how would bacteria survive such an onslaught? In addition to inhibiting the immune system, *B. burgdorferi* now appears to be able to take the form of what are called (a bit confusingly) "persister bacteria," like those found in certain hard-to-treat staph infections, which were long thought not to have existed in Lyme disease. Several researchers, including Ying Zhang at the Johns Hopkins Bloomberg School of Public Health and Kim Lewis at Northeastern University, have proposed that in Lyme these persister bacteria can enter a dormant state, allowing them to survive a normally lethal siege of antibiotics, which makes sense: Doxycycline functions not by directly killing bacteria but by inhibiting their replication. It affects only actively dividing bacteria, not dormant ones, relying on a healthy immune system to dispatch any *B. burgdorferi* that remain—something I had not understood until I spoke to Zhang. His findings offer a model for why some people would recover from Lyme and others could fail to clear the bacteria.

The big discovery, though, came when Zhang's team treated the mice with a three-antibiotic cocktail, including a drug known to work on per-sistent staph infections: the mice cleared the persistent *B. burgdorferi* infection. "We now have not only a plausible explanation but also a po-tential solution for patients who suffer from persistent Lyme-disease symptoms despite standard single-antibiotic treatment," Zhang told me.

Of course, even if active bacteria do remain in some Lyme patients, they may not be the cause of the symptoms. Paul Auwaerter, the clinical director of infectious diseases at Johns Hopkins School of Medicine and a former president of the IDSA, points out that Lyme bacteria can leave behind DNA debris that may trigger ongoing "low-grade inflamma-tory responses." In 2019, Lewis told me that the overarching question—"whether the pathogen is there and is slowly causing damage or has already left the body and has wrecked the immune system"—has yet to be settled, in his view. But, he said, "I'm optimistic that we and others are going to find a cure for PTLDS."

ON A BRISK MARCH DAY, I visited a research laboratory at Massa-chusetts General Hospital directed by Allen Steere, the rheumatologist who discovered Lyme disease and helped establish the testing parame-ters for it. A slim, gray-haired man with an intense gaze, he has be-come, in the eyes of many chronic Lyme patients, an embodiment of the medical system's indifference to their plight, because he has long sug-gested that many such patients were incorrectly diagnosed, and proba-bly never had Lyme disease in the first place. He has been shouted down at conferences and ambushed by people purporting to be journal-istic interviewers. Scientists who disagree with him had nonetheless singled him out to me for his commitment to studying Lyme. I wanted to hear his perspective on the disease and on the debate over chronic Lyme.

While underscoring that medicine can be humbling, and that Lyme disease is complex, Steere spoke with the calm air of someone setting a child straight. He emphasized, first, that in many people Lyme disease can resolve on its own without antibiotics. And then he carefully described a disease that in the United States frequently progresses through specific stages if untreated, beginning with an early rash and fever, followed by neurological symptoms, and culminating in inflammatory arthritis. The joint inflammation can continue for months or even years after antibiotic treatment, but not, he believes, because the bacteria persist. His research on patients who have these continuing arthritis symptoms has revealed one cause to be a genetic susceptibility to an ongoing inflammatory response. This discovery has led to effective treatment for the longer-term challenges of Lyme arthritis, using what are called "disease-modifying anti-rheumatic agents." It is also an important demonstration of one way that infections and genetics can collide to produce persistent inflammatory illness.

After I told him a little about my case, he struck a note of solicitous firmness. He told me that in his view, late-stage Lyme (which is what I had been diagnosed with) usually does not cause a lot of systemic symptoms, such as the fatigue and brain fog I had experienced. "I want you to free yourself from the Lyme ideology," he said. "You clearly were helped by antibiotic therapy. But I don't favor the idea that it was spirochetal infection. Of course, there are other infectious agents," he continued, noting that some of them trigger complex immune responses.

I left Steere's office unnerved, thinking that if I had met a doctor with some version of this view in 2014, I would never have started doxycycline and gotten better. But I was open to the idea that I had a condition other than Lyme that turned out to respond to antibiotics.

That night I curled up with my computer in my hotel room and reread a 1976 *New York Times* article about the discovery of Lyme disease. New things struck me, in particular the fact that at the time, Steere thought it was likely that Lyme was *not* a bacterial disease (as it in fact is), because the microorganism was not acting like a bacterium: "The bacterial infections that are known to cause arthritis leave permanent joint damage, and bacteria are easy to see in body fluids and easy to grow in test tubes. Every effort to culture bacteria from fluids and tissues from the patients has failed." Steere had moved on to a new possibility: "A virus is the most likely candidate," he told the *Times*. "Just because we haven't found one yet doesn't mean it isn't there. We'll keep looking." When I wrote to ask him if he had been fooled by Lyme disease back in the 1970s, he reminded me of how much he and others had learned in just a few years about this then-new infection. He went on to remind me that science can "lead to one 'dead end' after another. One needs to learn from these dead ends and continue trying."

"Anyone who says they really understand the pathophysiology of what's going on is oversimplifying to some degree," said Ramzi Asfour, a physician and member of the Infectious Diseases Society of America with notably open views on Lyme disease, when I reached him on the phone in his Bay Area office. Asfour has found that a one-size-fits-all approach to Lyme diagnosis and treatment is inadequate for most patients in his medical practice.

We do not know enough yet about diseases that are characterized by abnormal activity of the immune system, he emphasized. But alongside the usual standardized protocols, they clearly call for the tactics of personalized medicine because the immune system is so complex—and so individualized. Listening to patients is crucial. "Did you live in a moldy place? Are you chronically stressed?'" Asfour told me, illustrating the types of questions he asks patients. "I have a lot of patients I've been seeing for a year or two years who finally get better only after they realize they need to work on their nervous system." This complexity, Asfour says, is a problem for the conventional medical system.

"Being an infectious-disease doctor is usually pretty rewarding in the conventional sense," Asfour said. "The patient is in the ICU; you grow a bacterium, and you see it; then you give them a magic pill. They get better and walk home. It's very satisfying." The experience of Lyme patients challenges that model. "The conventional folks are very, very

good at what they do," Asfour continued. "But a patient with a constel-
lation of symptoms that doesn't clearly fit a diagnosis is not somebody
that they want to deal with." As the surgeon Atul Gawande wrote of
the medical profession, "Nothing is more threatening to who you think
you are than a patient with a problem you cannot solve."

AFTER EIGHT MONTHS OF on-and-off treatment, Dr. H decided that
I could stop taking antibiotics. It was the spring of 2015. In the white
space of the margins of this book lies the silence of all that I cannot put
into words. Suddenly I *knew* the life that I had lost in the years that I
had doubted my own perceptions. I felt like a person again, even if some
of the fatigue and dizziness of POTS and thyroid disease remained.
Those symptoms were manageable compared to the terrifying loss of
cognitive function that the Lyme had brought with it.

Sorrow rolled in and kept rolling.

Little webs of feeling that I'd ignored for years shivered in the breeze
of my wide-open mind.

SIXTEEN

FUTURITY

Antibiotics gave me my life back; I had never been more grateful for modern medicine. But I also knew that they wreak havoc on your gut, disrupting the balance of its bacteria. And so it was that in the fall of 2015, on an unseasonably hot September morning in England, I took a train from London's King's Cross Station to Hitchin, a town about thirty minutes north of London, where the Taymount Clinic was located, on a high street crowded with shops. (The clinic has since moved to a new location one stop up the line.) The clinic was founded in 2003 to help clients with digestive health issues and chronic illnesses. I checked in and waited on a cream-colored vinyl couch. The sweat on the back of my knees stuck to the cushion. Nervously, I studied the cluttered dark room, which felt nothing like an American medical office. In one corner stood a cabinet holding collagen bars and Bulletproof coffee.

I had flown across the Atlantic, traveled by train, and paid thousands of dollars to come to a clinic so that someone could inject me with other people's fecal matter. That's right: I was there to get what's called a "fecal microbiota transplant," or FMT. Once upon a time, you couldn't have paid me to do (or even contemplate) such a thing. But I wanted to get pregnant, and my research had left me with the sense that getting an FMT might help me recover from the months of damaging antibiotics I'd taken and possibly even reach a new level of health. As I sat there, though, confronted by the reality of what I was about to do, my brain was making excuses for backing out: *I don't need to do this; I'm not really sick anymore.*

If my Lyme diagnosis had unfolded tidily years earlier—with a tick bite, a bull's-eye rash, a quick round of antibiotics—I would never have found myself in England. But my years of searching for answers about why I felt sick all the time had fundamentally altered my relationship to medical science and to my body. I now understood that my sickness was probably a consequence of many complex intertwined factors, of which the Lyme infection was only one. And I had come to think that it was on me to protect my body, and to prevent disease, rather than just take drugs or search for a quick fix. Mounting evidence suggests that the microbiome is crucial to health and that damage to it can trigger everything from autoimmune disease to cancerous malignancies, as well as play a role in depression and anxiety. For people like me whose family history suggests a genetic tendency toward autoimmune disease, it is important to consider the role of the microbiome. I had spent years painstakingly following a diet designed to help restore microbiome health—fermented vegetables, yogurt, whole foods. But eight months of antibiotics had undone a lot of that work. My digestion was not what it had been. Even heaping amounts of kimchi and yogurt, I surmised, would not be enough to fix the damage wrought.

The idea to go to Taymount had actually come from Matt Galen, whom I had called when I was trying to decide whether to take antibiotics for Lyme or to try to treat the infection with herbs. Galen had told me, "Lyme is a nasty disease. Take the antibiotics; they are called for here. And when you're done, go get a fecal microbiota transplant from the Taymount Clinic in England—and you'll be almost as good as new." He gave me the clinic's contact information and explained to me why he felt their work was scientifically sound. The procedure was not cheap, but after doing some research, Jim and I agreed that the apparent benefits made it worth it. Of all the treatments I had tried, other than antibiotics, the FMT was likely to be the most significant (as well, of course, as being the most repulsive).

A woman in her forties with large brown eyes entered the waiting area and warmly introduced herself as Giovanna. "You must be Meghan! Come on back to the treatment room," she said. She had a remarkable broad smile, which I suspected was cultivated for the purpose of putting apprehensive clients at ease. In a small treatment room, furnished with a sink and a massage table, she introduced me to a young nursing assistant named Leila.

They explained what the procedure would entail: eight visits over two weeks during which I would receive, by enema, "samples" (I tried not to think too hard about this) collected from a host of donors who had been carefully screened for infections and pathogens after tests had determined that they were in possession of a healthy range of gut flora. They underscored that the donors had been fully screened, and that they had to be healthy and committed to eating a whole foods diet.

"The samples have been filtered so they're just the bacteria in solution. No food matter and no diseases. All clean and good," Leila said.

Was each day's sample from a different person? I asked.

"They're mixed together from a few people," Giovanna told me, "and you are going to get different samples, for diversity of microbiota."

Before any of that happened, though, I had to have a colonic—the colon needed to be as empty as possible to help the new gut flora establish themselves without resistance from the original compromised microbiome. As it began, Giovanna made relaxing small talk, chatting about travel plans and asking me questions about where I was staying. As the water pressure increased, debris from my intestines started to (as

Giovanna delicately put it) "release." It feels shameful the first time it happens. I made some excuse.

"We like dirty pipes!" Giovanna reassured me, laughing.

"Oh yes, this is a good release," Leila affably chimed in. "Exactly what we want to see, all the old stuff coming out."

I shut my eyes uncomfortably. As the colonic went on and on—time slows while other people are watching stool run out of you—Giovanna and Leila struck up a pleasingly banal conversation about how much they liked spending rainy days in their "jim-jams" (British for pajamas). I stared at the ceiling and pretended this wasn't happening. Eventually they turned off the water. It was time to get my sample.

I waited in silence on the table, heavily aware of the gown clutched around my naked hips, goose pimples speckling my thighs.

"Here are your babies!" Giovanna cried, opening the door. "Do you want to see?"

She was holding a kind of baster. I didn't want to look too closely.

"Wow," I said with faint enthusiasm. "So great!"

She came close, waving it at me. Leila instructed me to lie on my side. Then I felt a bit of pressure and a funny watery sensation I couldn't orient. And that was it.

"So you'll rest now with your knees up for thirty minutes," Giovanna said crisply. "We have a timer, and you'll change position every ten minutes. We find this helps people retain the implant better."

They left me alone. I looked around the bare room. I was on an exam table with a Bristol Stool Chart on the wall beside me. On the window ledge were two porcelain phrenology heads, staring implacably into the quiet air of the room.

THE IDEA THAT transferring fecal matter from one person to another via syringes might cure a host of difficult-to-treat diseases goes against everything I had learned as a child about germs and hygiene.

But, as we've seen earlier, today scientists understand that bacteria can be both harmful and good for us, and that the absence of balance among them can lead to illness, such as Crohn's or ulcerative colitis. (Various triggers can throw off the commensal—or beneficial—relationships among them.) A transplant helps treat those illnesses, it is theorized, by restoring a range of bacteria in the digestive tract. Our health is intimately tied to our bacteria: changes in our microbiome lead to changes in our immune system (and vice versa). Each of us is host to a colony of trillions, most of which live in our digestive tract. ("Our gut is home to more than 100 trillion bacteria," write the Stanford microbiologists Justin Sonnenburg and Erica Sonnenburg.) We inherit part of our microbiome from our mothers when we pass through the vaginal canal at birth, and from the early years we spend crawling on the floor and putting everything in our mouths. Much of the rest we get through food, by way of soil still attached to vegetables and fruits, for example. Certain foods, like bananas and sweet potatoes, contain loads of *prebiotics*—a kind of carbohydrate that feeds gut bacteria. One might think of prebiotics as probiotics' food; these nutrients help the good strains of microbes thrive and crowd out pathogens.

Over time, antibiotics and a Western diet high in processed foods have led to the extinction of whole species of microbiota in many people's guts. (One study found that healthy volunteers who took one week of antibiotics experienced significant changes to their microbiome for up to two years, including a notable decrease in variety of strains; exposure to antibiotics in infancy, another shows, leads to increased rates of asthma and weakened immune response.) Fewer strains of microbes lead to fewer chemical by-products made by those microbes—and those by-products, we are just beginning to understand, play a key role in modulating our immune system, turning on and off the cytokine signals that regulate immunity, impacting gene expression, and much more. "Without them, our immune system functions like a traffic system gone wild," one researcher told me.

When I first got sick, I had heard here and there about people who miraculously recovered from different bowel disorders following a fecal transplant. At that time, FMTs already had almost mythic status among chronically ill people as a miracle cure for all kinds of autoimmune disease and even depression and anxiety—a natural solution to the negative effects of an artificial modern life. But the procedure exploded in popularity sometime after 2013, when *The New England Journal of Medicine* published the stunning results of the first randomized controlled trial of a fecal microbiota transplant in the treatment of *Clostridium difficile* infections, which cause a serious case of diarrhea. The FMT was so effective, the researchers stopped the trial so that all patients in it could access the procedure. In 2012, graduate students at MIT founded a nonprofit "stool bank" called OpenBiome, at which they screen and freeze donor material to send to doctors and hospitals for use in FMTs. In 2014, the Cleveland Clinic deemed it one of the top medical innovations of the year. In 2016, the FDA stepped in, classifying stool as an investigational drug so that it could tightly regulate the procedure, limiting its common application to cases of *C. diff.* The alternative and the mainstream medical worlds had collided.

Accumulating medical evidence supports the theory that FMTs can be useful for far more than *C. diff* infections. The gut-brain axis that had sounded so outlandish to me when I first heard about it in 2012 is, we know today, key to human health. Gut bacteria influence serotonin and other neurotransmitters, researchers have found, raising questions about the role of our microbiome in predisposing us to a variety of illnesses. (Ninety percent of serotonin is made in the gut.) In 2010, a study published in *Neuroscience* found that rats given bifidobacteria (bacteria that aid in digestion) after being separated from their mothers persevered swimming in water longer, and had lower stress hormone levels, than those who had been given the SSRI citalopram. Studies in humans have had dramatic results. A neurobiologist at the University of

Oxford examined whether administering a prebiotic could modulate stress levels in humans. He gave some subjects galactooligosaccharide (GOS), a prebiotic that helps populate the gut with good bacteria, and others a placebo. The subjects who took the GOS had lower levels of cortisol and focused more on positive information than negative in a test in which words flashed quickly over a screen. A UCLA study of thirty-six female subjects found that those who ate yogurt containing probiotics twice a day for four weeks reacted more calmly to images of angry faces than subjects who did not, according to brain scans—the first study to document a connection between bacteria we eat and our brain function. Partial though these studies may be, they point to how powerfully our biome influences our well-being.

On Wednesday afternoon, the heat wave having finally broken and given way to a violent thunderstorm, I had my next-to-last treatment. Afterward, I met with Glenn and Enid Taylor, Taymount's founders. As rain lashed the windows, we talked in a large, orange-carpeted room in which two desks stood covered in papers; Enid, in a black skirt, sat at the desk opposite me. She interjected archly now and then, with a comedian's timing. Glenn was a charismatic, spry, lean man of about sixty with bright blue eyes and a shock of gray hair, who described himself early in our talk as "a renegade." (Despite his life's work, he was trained in engineering, and has taught himself much of what he knows about microbiology.)

"First, how is *your* treatment going?" Glenn asked, as I sat down on the couch. I told him I was feeling sick, and he said he thought that was a good sign—the critters were colonizing, in his phrasing.

As we chatted, Glenn and Enid explained how they came to administer FMTs at the clinic. At the time that they founded Taymount in 2003, the Taylors worked with patients who had gut flora dysbiosis. In

Glenn's view, gastroenterologists were paying too little attention to what their patients were experiencing. "Clearly any gastroenterologist will know his anatomy. But he doesn't understand the depths of the ocean," he told me. Glenn, by contrast, was very interested in the microbiome and what it was doing to his patients. Understanding that dysbiosis was caused by problems with the microbiome and gut inflammation, the clinic used colonics and probiotic suppositories to try to heal the gut. But he found that the procedures did not work as he had expected: the laboratory-bred probiotics did not colonize the gut well. He was unsure what to do next.

"This all started when a man called up Enid, actually," he said, and swiveled toward her.

"Oh dear, indeed it did," she said. "I got this call from a man asking if we did fecal transplants. I thought the idea was possibly a disgusting fetish. I hung up the phone and looked for as many ways to wipe off the handset as possible. 'You'll never guess what someone just asked me,' I told Glenn."

For Glenn, the call was a eureka moment. "I said, 'Ahh, *that's* how we do it. Give me that phone please!'"

He had realized that fecal transplants were the solution he had been looking for. As he explained, the lifespans of bacteria are very short, and they adapt quickly to whatever environment they find themselves in, including a lab. In our guts, bacteria have little hooks to help them hold on to intestinal walls and colonize. In a petri dish, they have no need to hold on to intestinal walls. Taylor realized they must be evolving away from the adaptations that help them stick to the intestines, and so with probiotics there was "no engraftment." In essence, the patients pooped them out before the bacteria could colonize and grow more of their strain.

I asked if this meant that probiotics—which I spent a lot of money on!—were a scam. No, he said. "They're very helpful, in fact. Having beneficial strains present affects the colonized strains for the better—they compete with the pathogenic strains and help push them out. But you have to keep taking them, which is a great business model." Taking probiotics is not going to change your microbiome long-term, in other words, but it can help you short-term, by temporarily introducing beneficial species.

After the man's call, Glenn became interested in the idea of a fecal microbiota transplant from a healthy person to a sick person. He studied how to do this in a manner that would not create problems for the recipient. Faced with skepticism, he thought back to the example of Barry Marshall, the scientist who proved *H. pylori* caused gastritis and ulcers by infecting himself with it. Taylor decided to do a self-implant. Finding that he had no negative side effects, he began treating patients in 2010. By 2021, the clinic had administered FMTs to around 3,750 people.

"Our understanding of the microbiome is still very partial," Taylor told me. "But it suggests the degradations to our biome are having a major effect on our health." This is because the bacteria are codependent—only one in eight strains can survive on its own—and if you lack that commensal community you may end up with gut dysbiosis. The problem with antibiotics is how broad they are—they strafe the entire gut, not just the dangerous strain, and change the delicate balance of power in the gut. "Medicine did this out of ignorance," Taylor said. "We thought that broad-spectrum antibiotics would always be sensible, because we'd get the pathogenic strain even if we were wrong in our diagnosis."

Bacteria can act differently in different people, depending on that community. Researchers I spoke to described this as "quorum sensing": with certain strains gone, other strains' gene expressions change, turning them from benign to malign. Shifts in our bacteria can also contribute to damage to the tight junctions of our intestinal barrier, the mucosal wall that allows us to absorb nutrients while preventing pathogens and food molecules from reaching the bloodstream. Gut dysbiosis can result in unsealed barriers and inflammatory responses. Food molecules escape into the blood, where the immune system responds to them, creating sensitivities—the so-called leaky gut syndrome discussed earlier. To heal, the gut barrier needs to be rebuilt with tighter junctions, which the FMT helps with.

The effects of an FMT are so strong that some gastroenterologists believe we should start treating certain infections and digestive disorders by trying to rebuild the gut wall with FMTs *instead of* using antibiotics, even if FMTs are slower to take effect. (One person told me that the peak beneficial effects seem to occur four months to two years after the procedure.)

In the meantime, Taylor told me that he believes that diet and antibiotics are partly responsible for growing rates of immune-mediated illness. "For millions of years, until very recently," he said, "most of the environment for the gut was stable, based on a hunter-gatherer diet. Our food changed geographically and seasonally at a manageable rate. Very suddenly, in the nineteenth century, we changed that when we industrialized food. In the twentieth century, we said, 'We don't even need food, we can use chemicals.'" That change upended our microbiome, because bacteria evolve much faster than we do; some species reproduce every six minutes. And so, he said, "We can't keep up with how to survive our new microbiomes."

Today, we still are in the dark about a great deal of what the microbiome does. "We don't really know how our immune system and bacteria fully interact," Glenn continued. "What if our immune system is partially a system by which we interact with our microbiome? What if," he said suddenly, waggling his fingers, "the microbacteria are *interlocutors* for the immune system? They are our interlocutors, and the conversation has gone awry."

I brought up some of the claims I had seen made on behalf of

FMTs—that they were the frontier of a new kind of medicine and could reverse all kinds of chronic health conditions. Glenn was circumspect. "We ignored the microbiome for years," he said. "And now we want to use it to try to normalize the human gut. But what *is* normal?" He ruffled his soft white hair and smiled.

"We know that we *don't* know. That's the key." He paused. "FMT is not necessarily the twenty-first-century panacea to all ills."

THE CLINIC HAD WARNED ME in advance that I might feel tired and have flu-like symptoms after my treatment, but I had discounted the severity of the side effects. By the end of the first week, I felt as though I had the worst flu I'd ever had. My exhaustion was profound. On day four, I could barely walk from the clinic to the train. On day six—the first day of the second week—I started feeling achy and feverish. My hips throbbed.

Annie, a nutritionist at the clinic, came to give me a post-FMT dietary plan: lots of prebiotics (to feed the new bacteria inside me), vegetables, and high-quality meat such as grass-fed beef. I was to avoid processed food, sugar, and coffee, which often carries mold on it or is treated with pesticides. (If coffee was necessary—it was!—they recommended Dave Asprey's Bulletproof coffee, which is formulated to be mold-free.) Annie told me the new microbes would slowly colonize my gut, leading to long-term change. Some patients ended up able to eat foods to which they once were intolerant, but she cautioned me not to expect as much: this was uncommon. Still, she hoped, I would feel more energetic, less bloated, less given to inflammatory responses.

The next morning, I had chills and a fever. I called my nutritionist in the United States to tell her how sick I felt. Should I be concerned? She said, "Look, it makes sense—you effectively just had an organ transplant."

I emailed Annie to say I didn't know that I could finish the treatment; I was having a powerful immune reaction to it. She told me not to worry—lots of folks managed to do only five treatments. I could return for the rest on a future visit. Then she wished me luck.

On the train to the airport from London, a massive double rainbow broke out across the sky, arching down behind the outer suburbs. I was returning home to try to get pregnant. I decided to take it as an omen.

EIGHT WEEKS LATER, more energetic than I had been in years, I got pregnant. I was thirty-nine. In the early, dizzying weeks of conceiving after years of trying and failing, I felt many forms of metaphysical joy, but the pregnancy, I believed, was a story I had to work to hold in my mind. If I didn't, it might fade away, like a dream you can't remember after you wake up.

At night I listened to a meditation track and visualized a white light entering my body, calming my immune system, because I didn't trust my body to do anything right. At night, I dreamed, too, about old memories and things I had seen when I was young. The images were preverbal and sense drenched: red rooms, peacock-feathered pillows, the distinctive brown-palm velour wallpaper in (I think) my first pediatrician's brownstone office. I saw my mother, too, her belly large as she lay on the couch, pregnant with my brother. I woke up sweating, and in the dark her face seemed to float near mine. Superstitiously, the idea flashed in my mind that the baby inside me had been hiding out with my mother, waiting to arrive.

I had something known as "antiphospholipid antibodies," which the rheumatologist Michael D. Lockshin had identified as a threat to some pregnancies. I also had other autoimmune markers that could perhaps lead to immunological complications in pregnancy. My doctor put me on steroids and infusions of something called "intravenous immunoglobulins," which is a collection of other people's antibodies, to help prevent my dysfunctional immune system from accidentally harming the fetus.

Other than requiring these interventions, I had an uneventful pregnancy. The baby just grew and grew, as babies are supposed to. I marveled at what it was like to live at last in a body that worked. Women with POTS and autoimmune diseases can feel much better while pregnant, in fact; I was one of them. I remained uncertain and anxious, but as the pregnancy went on the feeling evolved. My body had failed me; my body was now not failing me. Perhaps all along my idea of failure had been wrong. Perhaps my body had been working hard to keep me as well as it could despite a serious, life-altering infection, and I needed to find a new story about it. A story that allowed for the contingency of identity, of health, of hope. One that saw survival of any kind as a form of strength. What I had experienced *was* life itself, the body straining to survive despite the odds stacked against it.

In the summer of 2016, I gave birth to a baby, a boy—C. He arrived curled like the letter, screaming and then curious. His entrance into my life brought joy and exhaustion.

SEVENTEEN

UNCERTAINTY

Real dangers attend the contested realities of Lyme disease and other tick-borne illnesses. The summer that C was born, my father began to suffer drenching night sweats, fatigue, and aches and pains. His tests were negative for Lyme but suggestive of ehrlichiosis, another tick-borne infection, and his doctor—in the heart of Lyme country—decided to treat what seemed like a plausible culprit and its co-infection. My father was put on doxycycline. He didn't improve, which surprised me, given that I had seen near-immediate results. Then one day in late October, when my son was two months old, my brother found my father at home, on the verge of collapse, and took him to an ER, where batteries of tests revealed that he had a different problem. He was suffering from stage 4 Hodgkin's lymphoma. It had progressed stealthily while he was being treated for an infection he might not have had.

Visiting him in the hospital, I was stunned by how frail he was. I couldn't help wondering how much those lost months might have cost him, as the cancer advanced and weakened him—all because Lyme had seemed like a plausible explanation, and we still don't have diagnostic technologies that can dependably sort out whether or not you have a tick-borne disease.

Unable to care for himself, my father came to live with me, Jim, and our son in our apartment in Brooklyn while he underwent chemotherapy. He moved in a few days after Thanksgiving. The months that followed were harrowing, hectic processions of visits to the doctor, calls to the insurance company, and searches for food that might appeal to a finicky patient. There were weeks where I never sat down by myself: I was either helping my father or caring for my baby. C wasn't sleeping through the night, nor was my father. The first night he spent with us, he fell badly while trying to use the bathroom. I slept lightly, part of my brain listening for cries from either of the two. Caregiver to the generations bracketing me, I began to feel achy and bone tired. My father started chemo. Slowly, his cancer retreated, and he improved enough to move back to Connecticut, where my brothers found a caretaker to cook and drive him to and from his last few chemo appointments.

My father's experience dramatically illustrated the cost of the decades of uncertainty about Lyme disease and its diagnostic criteria, including the limited research and the lack of funding. For my father, the Lyme diagnosis masked the more serious and appropriate diagnosis of advanced cancer. For me, it got me to a long-overdue essential treatment—but what ailed me could not be reduced to just Lyme disease, as it sometimes is in the case of people with medically unexplained symptoms who ultimately receive a Lyme diagnosis. I was lucky that my Lyme doctor was alert to this; he was the first to point out that I had other issues, such as POTS and autoimmune disease, and he did not attribute all my symptoms to the persistence of tick-borne illness. Openly acknowledging how little we understand of the immunological aftermath of infections is key not only to thinking about tick-borne illness, but also to how we think about conditions like long COVID, ME/CFS, and autoimmune disease, so that we may begin to develop the much-needed and long overdue tools to tease apart, identify, and ultimately treat such conditions.

OVER THE YEARS, I'VE SPENT a lot of time thinking about both my father's story and my own. And I always end at the same place: Whatever ends up being the truth of chronic Lyme disease, the IDSA's dismissive approach to patients did not help its cause and in some ways set the stage for chronic Lyme to become a dug-in point of contestation. In responding to patients' descriptions of ongoing symptoms by emphasizing that such symptoms are common in the general population, it invalidated the urgent reality of these symptoms and silenced patients' testimony. What the IDSA long seemed unwilling to acknowledge is that patients were coming to them with their own knowledge. Indeed, just because a symptom is common—and subjective—does not mean that a patient cannot tell the difference between a normal version of it and a pathological one, the way we experience the difference in severity between the common cold and the flu.

I have experienced both normal fatigue and pathological fatigue, which is altogether different from tiredness or physical exhaustion. It is a feeling that my body's most essential energy functions have screeched to a halt. I suspect I understand the language of illness more intimately than do many of the researchers who study disease; I am a native speaker, you might say. For me and others who have been seriously ill, the idea that we could confuse these symptoms with the normal aches and pains of life is laughable. When I was very ill, I could barely walk down the block, and fatigue blacked out whole days; it felt as if my body were made of sand, and as if molasses had invaded my brain.

By contrast, today as I write, my joints hurt, my brain is a little foggy, and I'm tired. But these I take to be something closer to the normal aches and pains of daily life. *These* are the kinds of subjective symptoms the CDC and the IDSA deem common. They distract me, but I can sit and write and make lunch for my children and enjoy—*experience*—my life. I am present. I am, more or less, me. That is not how I felt when I was sick. I imagine anyone who knew me well in my midthirties, when I was at my sickest, could tell that there was nothing I wanted more than to realize the promise of my own still-young life. This is the real tragedy of our cultural psychologization of diseases we don't understand: the ways such dismissals leave patients to suffer alone, their condition turned into a character flaw.

After I'd been on antibiotics for a few months, people would ask if I was "better." I was in fact better, but not in the way they meant: I still was dealing with health issues every day. I still broke out in weird rashes and was, at times, inexplicably tired. I still couldn't eat certain foods—gluten and eggs, mainly—without getting headaches and feeling groggy for a day. But mostly I nodded and smiled. I knew that to talk about Lyme as a chronic condition was to put at risk my standing as a reliable narrator of my own experience. All I knew was that taking antibiotics had led to a turning point in my health.

Even so, I remained haunted by what I didn't know about my own illness. One of the strange things about finding that the antibiotics worked was that I had to shift my illness narrative yet again. First, I had thought nothing was wrong with me: I was just sensitive. Then, I had thought I had a thyroid disease I could take a pill for and get better from. Then, I thought that a still-undiagnosed autoimmune disease was making me sick. And then, I had come to think that tick-borne infections had caused at least some of my symptoms. I *now* had to decide if I thought it was an active infection that was continuing to make me sick, or the aftereffects of immune dysregulation (or both). In this sense, the possibility that I had one or more long-standing undiagnosed tick-borne infections brought more, not less, uncertainty with it.

And so the things I learned while treating my illness as an autoimmune disease had not been a waste of my time. Of course, I still had plenty of autoimmune markers in my lab work; the antibiotics had not solved everything. I still experienced some fatigue, brain fog, and memory issues. In one of our appointments, Dr. H said, "You'll never know if the autoimmunity made the Lyme worse or if the Lyme brought on autoimmune issues earlier than they might have developed, had you not been bitten by a tick."

In this sense, PTLDS, autoimmunity, ME/CFS, and long COVID are diseases of our era, conditions that illuminate the need for a shift in medical thinking, from the model of the specific disease entity with a clear-cut solution to the messy reality shaped by both infection and genetics and our whole social history, a reality that no one yet fully understands. In the absence of certainty, medical science remains unsure what story to tell. Too often it turns away from patients rather than listening to the long and chaotic stories we tell, narratives that start and stop and double back, searching for meaning in the peculiar rash that broke out that day or the car accident that triggered pain or the death after which nothing was the same.

Indeed, one reason that people who may or may not have Lyme disease cling to the diagnosis of chronic Lyme as a name for their medically unexplained symptoms is that the impersonal nature of modern medicine has no better explanations, at least not on the level of storytelling. When we suffer, we want recognition. Where science is silent, narrative creeps in.

Part Three

HEALING

EIGHTEEN

SILENCE AND HEALING

What does it mean for a chronically ill patient to heal? In some cases, it may mean a remission of disease. But in others, it means the patient is now able to manage the illness with some degree of integrity. In order to tell the true story of my illness and the Lyme diagnosis, I have to describe the setbacks, the many ups and downs that were part of being sick. In the spring of 2017, four months into my father's chemotherapy, when C was eight months old, my interlude of feeling energetic and mostly symptom-free abruptly ended. In early April, we both got sick with a virus, and I didn't recover. The usual started up again: My body ached. My brain got foggy. C wasn't yet sleeping through the night, but my fatigue was the result of more than sleep deprivation. Flickers of electric shocks—*Oh no*—began to shoot along my legs. My primary care doctor found that the Epstein-Barr virus was active in my system again, and I had high autoimmune titers. I was exhausted, unwell, and snappish. It was once again challenging to teach or to write.

By June, my father had made an almost full recovery from the cancer, or so it seemed. Later we would learn that the chemo had taken a profound toll on his heart. But my body didn't bounce back. With a frail father, a one-year-old, and a body recovering from illness, I was drained. In August, I drove up to see Dr. Horowitz again. Based on my labs, he suggested that the Lyme infection had recurred and that I needed another course of antibiotics. I hesitated. I still wasn't sure whether to believe that the bacteria could persist in my body after months of antibiotics, and I attributed my ill health to an autoimmune flare or postviral fatigue. I was scheduled at the end of the month to take a work trip to Seattle. At Jim's urging, I decided to visit Washington's Olympic National Park, in the hope that a brief rest would help me feel better.

THE OLYMPIC NATIONAL PARK STRETCHES down coastal Washington and east toward Seattle on a thumb of land known as the Olympic Peninsula, some sixty miles long by ninety miles wide. About a three-hour ride by car from Seattle, it feels much farther away. Within it are volcanic beaches scattered with the remains of massive Sitka spruces; evergreen-crowded mountains; broad, flat valleys; and the Hoh Rain Forest, through which twelve miles of hiking trails and the glacier-formed Hoh River run. One of the quietest places in the country, it is home to what may be the most complex ecosystem in the United States.

It was an unusually warm and sunny day in August when I arrived. I was walking the grounds of my hotel in Kalaloch Beach, an hour's drive from the rain forest, when I heard another guest call out, "Do you want to see some whales?"

I climbed up into the gazebo beside him and looked where he was pointing. A delicate spout of water breached the air over the vast ocean. And then—a fin of an orca arcing over a wave.

"They've been feeding all day," he said.

Down at the beach, the dark gray sand was velvety and warm. I walked past dead jellyfish and oyster shells and the slender bones of seagulls. Before me was nothing but ocean—no ships, no airplanes, no buildings. The noise of the ocean was so huge and steady it felt like a silence in its own right. An orca lifted itself out of the water, baring its smooth back, and for a moment I felt its weight settle on me.

Being alone allowed me to reflect on how much had happened in the past two years of slow recovery, the kind of recovery that had brought pleasure and possibility back into my life but that had not made me "better" in the traditional sense of the word. Though the sun was strong, mist clung to a distant headland, like a scene from an Emily Brontë novel. In the quiet, all the thoughts that noise had held at bay rushed in. Here, announcing themselves, were my shock at my father's illness, the exhaustion at the insistent reality of my new son. And the almost impossible grief I still felt about my mother, who had died almost ten years earlier and would never know C. I thought about all that he would lose by not knowing her. I climbed atop a mound of beach logs—enormous spruces, some fifty feet long, piled up like matchsticks by the roaring ocean—and let the driftwood warm my feet, and the silence pool in my ears, and the sorrow sit. My quest to find answers about what was happening in my body had taken me far away from standard medical appointments and deep into meditations on what a life should be like, how wounds could be healed, and what to do when they can't be.

As much as we want silence, we also work hard to blot it out. Adrift in noise and bustle, we duck confrontation with the metaphysical and the existential. We avoid the enduring regret at how we treated an old, estranged friend, the fear that our life has been a project of self-delusion—that its gilded hand-stitched brocade may in fact be moth-eaten. Who wants to think about all that, really?

But sitting there I thought, too, about the fact that some kinds of healing can be so slow you barely notice them.

. . .

"THE IDEA THAT PHYSICAL SPACE might contribute to healing does, it turns out, have a scientific basis," Esther M. Sternberg notes in *Healing Spaces: The Science of Place and Well-Being*. A 1984 study, published in *Science*, found that when hospital rooms have windows with a view of something natural, patients heal more rapidly than they do without one: the environmental psychologist Roger Ulrich examined hospital records of forty-six patients who had gallbladder surgery between 1972 and 1981, and who had had different views out their window. One group had windows overlooking a grove of trees. The other group looked out at a brick wall. The patients overlooking the trees left the hospital almost a full day earlier than the other patients, and needed less pain medication.

Before the technological advances of the twentieth century, medicine had often believed that environment played a role in healing. In ancient Greece, temples of healing were located far from busy towns, some overlooking the sea. In the Middle Ages and Renaissance, too, homes of healing were often beautiful, such as the Hospices de Beaune, one of the most handsome buildings in the city of Beaune, France, which was built as a hospital for the indigent. In the nineteenth century, tuberculosis sanatoriums prioritized clean, dry air at high altitudes and lots of sunlight. Many nineteenth-century clinics and hospitals included a large solarium (from the Latin *sol*, "sun"), in which patients could sit and absorb sunlight as they healed.

In the late nineteenth century, a Danish scientist named Niels Finsen posited that sunshine played a role in health and healing, especially for those with chronic illnesses such as lupus vulgaris, a form of cutaneous tuberculosis. Growing up in Denmark, he was thought to be rather slow; a rector at his school wrote, "Niels was a very nice boy, but his gifts were small and he was quite devoid of energy." Finsen was eventually diagnosed with an inherited metabolic disorder called Niemann-Pick disease. He later wrote that his illness was "responsible" for his research: "I suffered from anaemia and tiredness, and since I lived in a house facing the north, I began to believe that I might be helped if I received more sun. I therefore spent as much time as possible in its rays. As an enthusiastic medical man I was of course interested to know *what benefit* the sun really gave."

Finsen was able to show that skin lesions from smallpox and tuberculosis improved with phototherapy, due to the stimulating (and possibly bactericidal) effects on skin cells. His work on lupus vulgaris led him to be awarded the Nobel Prize in 1903 for his development of a novel therapeutic process using concentrated ultraviolet light. When a doctor named Auguste Rollier, inspired by Finsen, began to champion heliotherapy, light therapy took off. In 1903, Rollier opened the first sunlight clinic, where patients were gradually exposed to more and more sun until they grew healthy.

At the start of the twentieth century, the sun was invited into hospitals; by the end of it, the sun had been pushed out of them. "By the late twentieth century, state-of-the-art hospitals were generally designed to accommodate state-of-the-art equipment," Sternberg observes in *Healing Spaces*. "Often, the hospital's physical space seemed meant to optimize care of the equipment rather than care of the patients." "To optimize care of the equipment": I recalled how in my surgery for endometriosis, I'd been wheeled into a freezing cold room, where I waited for hours, hungry and shivering, before the operation got under way. "The machines do better in this temperature," a nurse told me, kindly offering me a heated blanket.

THE WORLD HEALTH ORGANIZATION's definition of healing goes beyond the mere curing of disease. It defines health as "a state of complete physical, mental, and social well-being and not merely the absence of disease or infirmity." If we want to think about the ways medicine can do better, we will need to engage with this definition—especially when it comes to chronic illness. If doctors want to help patients heal, they need to take into consideration the things that contribute to a person's sense of well-being, whether it is sunlight, quiet, nature, or something else entirely. Sternberg reports she once asked Ann Berger, the chief of the Pain and Palliative Care Service at the NIH Clinical Center, for her definition of healing. Berger replied, "In palliative care, healing is thought of as a sense of wholeness. It is not being cured necessarily, but feeling whole." A patient is healed, that is, not solely by steroids or antibiotics, but also by nature, thrilling conversation, touch, empathy—being made to feel whole, rather than distraught, as she exits doctors' appointments.

Paradoxically, during the time I was sick, I became "less inwardly focused than communally aware," as George Prochnik puts it in his book *In Pursuit of Silence*, describing the effect of a Quaker meeting he once attended. My time as a person living with an unidentified illness tore off the private mask that isolated me. It left a reminder in me that the bell tolls for all of us, that my predicament is your predicament, and your predicament mine, because I am implicated in it.

John Donne wrote his famous line "No man is an island" after almost dying from spotted fever (thought to be typhus) during an outbreak in 1623. Donne was fifty-one and the dean of St. Paul's Cathedral. His daughter was engaged to be married when he became gravely ill. He urged her to wed while he was in the hospital so he could be sure that she would be taken care of. From his bed, he listened to the church bells around him toll not only weddings but the many deaths from the epidemic.

Physically, Donne felt alone, as he writes in *Devotions upon Emergent Occasions*, a twenty-three-part prose work about his illness. "Variable, and therefore miserable condition of man! this minute I was well, and am ill, this minute," he reflects, meditating on the uncertain night land of illness. "I am surprised with a sudden change, and alteration to worse, and can impute it to no cause, nor call it by any name." This uncertainty initially brings with it an almost unbearable sense of isolation: "As sickness is the greatest misery, so the greatest misery of sickness is solitude." And yet from the loneliness of his hospital bed, as he listened to funeral and wedding bells ring around him, he came to his famous insight about the spiritual connectedness of human experience: "No man is an island, entire of itself; every man is a piece of the continent, a part of the main. . . . Any man's death diminishes me, because I am involved in mankind, and therefore never send to know for whom the bells tolls; it tolls for thee."

One does not have to be Christian to see that Donne was right. To be ill is to recognize this interconnectedness—to understand how much we are "a part of the main." But to be ill in America today is to be brought up against the pathology of a culture that denies this fact. In the worst moments of my illness, I was alone because of the ways that we have allowed ourselves to believe that the self, rather than community, must do all the healing.

A FEW MONTHS LATER, after going back on antibiotics—which got rid of the worst of my symptoms within days—I got pregnant with my second son. The pregnancy was rough in the usual ways—morning sickness, discomfort—and because I got very anemic. But after the doctor sent me for three iron infusions early in my second trimester, I felt good for the remainder of the pregnancy—in some ways more energetic than ever. It was as if having more circulating blood cells flushed me with health. I looked less wan, too. Jim commented on it one night. "It finally looks like you have enough color in your face," he said.

I gave birth to R, my second son, that July. With two children less than two years old, my days and nights became a blur of exhaustion and joy, spit-up and blear. The old symptoms crowded back—brain fog, body aches, a fatigue that never left—and teaching was once more a challenge I could barely meet. But this time I knew that there was a path, somehow. Three years earlier, these symptoms threatened my sense of possibility: children, work, a life as a writer. Today, they depressed me, but I knew more about what was causing them and why and what might or might not help me get back to a baseline that allowed me to function. And besides, here was the futurity I had wanted: the baby's dark eyes studying mine as he nursed, his plump, plush hand curling around my pinky finger, while beside us on the rug his brother built a Magna-Tile castle, turrets and spikes galore. My life might still be circumscribed, and ringed by sometimes debilitating fatigue and pain, but I was acutely aware of how lucky I was to have recovered even this much. I hoped that it would stay this way for long enough for my kids to remember me as a mother who once could run along the beach with them.

NINETEEN

SOLUTIONS

Your suffering is burdensome to me," my friend J, a moral and legal philosopher, told me, rhetorically, at dinner on a chilly Monday night in January. It was my birthday. A historic snowstorm was about to hit the Northeast. On television the newscasters had been cautioning that the storm would last two full days and leave a snowfall of memorable proportions. A group of my neighbors and I had gone out in search of flashlights and batteries and wine before the weather closed us into our apartments. The snow was already coming down briskly, softly coating the world outside the window.

J and I had turned, in our conversation, to the subject of everyday injustices, of the sort that whole groups of people regularly experience. I had asked whether it constituted an injustice when a doctor or a friend failed to believe that a sick person really was sick. I wanted to know why, in his view of human character, it appears to be difficult for doctors (and the rest of us) to recognize suffering that we cannot name— why we are so quick to think a person is exaggerating or faking it? What is behind this refusal to recognize suffering?

"Even if doctors don't know what to *do*," I said, "and even if the lab tests are inconclusive, why not accept the testimony of the patient? Why do we have a system that's so quick to distrust the very people it serves?"

"Well," he said, "recognizing your suffering puts a burden on me."

"But all I'm talking about is recognition. There's no course of treatment to be done, let's say; no medical consequence."

"Think about it," he continued. "Just the *act* of recognizing you are ill makes a claim on me, doesn't it? I have to respond. I have to empathize. And that takes a toll on me. And the more people I have to empathize with, the harder it is. When you're sitting in front of me and suffering—not you," he said, as if he could see that I was beginning to take his words personally, "but anybody—it really does make a claim on the person being asked to recognize it."

Even something as simple as recognition is a burden, J argued, if the witness to illness is not prepared—if the witness has nothing to offer, or if he or she is emotionally drained.

That there is energy involved in the act of recognition was, I realized, true, and its truth was a problem for those who were ill. As the literary critic Hermione Lee writes in her introduction to Virginia Woolf's *On Being Ill*, "The world can't afford regular sympathy; it would take up the whole working day." Woolf, explaining why literature speaks so much of the mind, writes, "Those great wars which the body wages with the mind a slave to it, in the solitude of the bedroom against the assault of fever or the oncome of melancholia, are neglected. Nor is the reason far to seek. To look these things squarely in the face would need the courage of a lion tamer; a robust philosophy; a reason rooted in the bowels of the earth."

But this is what we need. We need a restorative whole-being approach that goes beyond what the current medical system typically offers the chronically ill patient. And we also need structural reform and a commitment to research. On a warm fall day, I met the economist David Cutler at his office at Harvard in an imposing marble building whose halls were lined with black-and-white photos of famous economists. We talked about the structural and economic difficulties of chronic-illness care.

"We know that when doctors work more closely with their patients they get better outcomes," Cutler said. "For example, if you take the diabetics who are not coming in for their HbA1c testing"—a test that measures one's average level of blood sugar over the past three months—"or their cholesterol screening or whatever, if the nurse calls them with a reminder and says, 'David, you haven't been in, you're supposed to come in every three months, it's been four months, would you like to schedule an appointment for Thursday afternoon?' then people will come in. It's not rocket science: it's basic block-and-tackle outreach."

The question is how we can structure incentives for medicine to do that. "What we know is that if you make it the default to do the right thing, people will do better," he said, noting that American health care lacked most of the necessary infrastructure. "The industry I often compare chronic disease to is financial planning. People pay Fidelity and Vanguard a lot of money. What they're paying them for is the convenience of making it easy to save for retirement. But no one has really invented that for health planning in cases like chronic illness, because it turns out that financial planning is easier," he said.

I asked Cutler why no one seemed to be organizing and managing care, offering advice about how to manage illnesses that seem to respond to sleep, diet, and so forth.

"Doctors are not trained to do this," Cutler said. "A doctor is trained like a tradesman. A surgeon is trained to cut you open, a plumber is trained to fix your pipes, a dermatologist is trained to check your skin. They're not trained to manage you. So someone has to step into that role. That's the biggest missing thing in health care, in part because the economics don't work, or haven't worked. What always strikes me: Who are the three highest paid people on the football team? The quarterback, the left tackle—the person who protects the quarterback from the blind side—and the coach. What the hell is the coach getting paid for? He never touches the ball during the game. He's not very fit. But he's bringing everything together. He's *paid* to bring all this together.

"No one does this for your health. When I had cats, the veterinarian would call or send a note saying, 'Time to bring your cats in.' The dentist does that. But not the doctor. They feel like they don't need the patients.

"The question is," he continued, "doctors are not trained to do any of this, so how are they going to do it? They don't have any management training, they don't have any economics training, they don't have any sales training."

Susan Block, the Harvard palliative care pioneer, pointed out that in many places, communication-skills training in medicine is "primitive." But there are successes. Recent advances in geriatric medicine and palliative care embody what can happen when the U.S. medical system shifts from high-tech intervention (which can bring its own problems) to helping patients *live with* their condition. Geriatric and palliative care doctors are trained to elicit patients' own attitudes about what matters most to them. Medical schools are also trying to reform medicine's longstanding habit of patient blaming. Some—not enough, Block implied—are putting more effort into teaching students key communication skills.

Communication skills clearly aren't enough, though. A lot of people with autoimmune diseases would like to see the establishment of clinical autoimmune centers, where a single doctor would coordinate a patient's care, as at a cancer center. In Israel, the Sheba Medical Center established a Center for Autoimmune Diseases, where the doctors take a functional medicine approach to health and have established a more coordinated model than is often seen in the United States. One hopes more changes will follow. In the United States, the West Penn Hospital in Pittsburgh, Pennsylvania, in collaboration with the Autoimmune Association, opened the Allegheny Health Network (AHN) Autoimmunity Institute in 2018. The institute is a center for coordinated auto-immune care run by Joseph Ahearn, a rheumatologist specializing in lupus, and overseen by Susan Manzi, who is also director of AHN's Lupus Center of Excellence, which provided the inspiration for the Au-toimmunity Institute, an umbrella organization that includes multiple centers. As Ahearn told me, "The goal was to take the lupus model and blast it out for all autoimmune disease. We realized you could have a center for excellence for as many diseases as we could support, and that you didn't have to have silos. You could use the same teams for multiple autoimmune diseases."

The Autoimmunity Institute has the aspirational sound of a new venture: billing itself as "the first of its kind in the world," the institute promises "a new approach to autoimmune disease care." It offers same-day, in-depth appointments with doctors across seventeen disciplines and prides itself on its streamlined coordination of care. Physicians may spend hours talking to patients and one another. In planning the insti-tute, Ahearn asked for an open work plan with space for the doctors and nurses to "huddle" after seeing patients, where they share insights and communicate about treatment plans in real time. The institute holds a weekly multidisciplinary conference in which, Ahearn told me, "We are talking about cases rare as hen's teeth, ones you can't find in the literature"—say, a patient with lupus autoantibodies, "who also has skin changes that suggest scleroderma and a pulmonary lesion on a lung X-ray"—and the doctors talk it out together. On the research front, the institute invests in cutting-edge attempts to create better diagnostic tools (such as "liquid biopsies," Ahearn said) while the clinical arm aims "not to put patients into diagnostic boxes, because we know our cur-rent diagnostic criteria are imperfect. We will sometimes say, 'We don't know *what* you have, we're not going to put a label on it, but this is how we are going to treat you, based on what we see.'" When I got acutely sick, I could only dream of such a scenario! Instead, I laboriously made my many appointments, trundling from doctor to doctor, trying to get them to share information and offer treatments.

Encouragingly, new technologies are allowing innovative researchers to pursue answers that weren't available to us before. Two things make Amy Proal, the PolyBio Research Foundation microbiologist, cautiously hopeful about the future of research into ME/CFS, long COVID, and other infection-associated illnesses: scientists are now looking for pathogens in tissues, not just in blood, and they are doing it with better technology. "The technologies and tools we have had to identify pathogens in patients have been very limited," she explained. "And we are beginning to better understand that the pathogens rarely persist in fluids; many of these infections are caused by organisms that preferentially infect the nervous system. To me, what is going to blow open the field is that we can now use advanced methods to look for organisms in the blood and *tissues* of patients. We are starting autopsy work that can actually look at patients' tissues and brains and the central nervous system where pathogens wreak the most havoc. And we are doing it with tech that is vastly better than even what we had five years ago."

Such innovative research is leading to fresh insights into the ways that the immune system, pathogens, and our microbes are engaged in a dance that may affect our metabolism, our moods, or even the production of cancerous tumors. The door is opening to novel ways of thinking about disease. The question is whether the will is now there to understand what causes long-stigmatized diseases like ME/CFS.

THERE MAY BE REASONS FOR a patient like me to hope that meaningful change is not too far off. If the coronavirus pandemic has brought any hope with it, it is that the scope of long COVID leaves us poised for a paradigm shift in how we think and talk about chronic, system-roaming, immune-mediated diseases. As devastating as COVID has been to the world, one effect of the pandemic has been to shine a light on chronic illness in a way that may bring help to those who have been overlooked for much too long. The very magnitude of the pandemic has made the impact of COVID's long-term effects unignorable. Funding is newly available; the need for research is evident. During the pandemic, many academic medical hospitals set up post-COVID care centers in a quest to help the growing numbers of patients with what has come informally to be called long COVID and, more formally, "post-acute COVID syndrome." In some ways, the pace of progress has been remarkable. Looked at in the most hopeful light, it suggests that Western medicine may finally reckon openly with similar contested illnesses, even as we still face a crisis of as-yet-unknown proportions that may change the future of millions of Americans.

The quest at Mount Sinai's Center for Post-COVID Care—one of the first such centers in the United States—began with a mystery. During the first wave of the coronavirus pandemic in New York City in the spring of 2020, Zijian Chen, an endocrinologist, turned to an online survey of COVID-19 patients who were more than a month past their initial infection but still experiencing symptoms. Because COVID-19 was thought to be a two-week respiratory illness, Chen anticipated that he would find only a small number of people who were still sick. That's not what he saw. "I looked at the number of patients that were in the database and it was, I think, eighteen hundred patients," he told me. "I freaked out a little bit. *Oh my god, there's so many patients telling us that they still have symptoms.*" A realization dawned on him: America was not simply struggling to contain a once-in-a-century pandemic. Many patients were, for unknown reasons, not recovering. Startlingly, most had had mild cases of COVID-19. Yet they were reporting significant ongoing symptoms—"shortness of breath, heart palpitations, chest pain, fatigue, and brain fog," Chen told me.

Chen quickly convened a multidisciplinary group of doctors at the

Center for Post-COVID Care to help patients manage their ongoing symptoms. He also partnered with unconventional thinkers like David Putrino, the director of rehabilitation innovation for the Mount Sinai Health System—a clinician who spends his time on questions that many doctors don't think about, including "measuring things that are hard to measure," as he told me. Mount Sinai had brought Putrino in to help it think outside the box about how it practiced rehabilitative medicine. He often gathers specialists in groups, to counter the American health care system's signature mode—"everything is very hyperspecialized, and professionals don't speak to one another," as he put it.

The center began triaging patients with ongoing symptoms, referring them to specialists and teasing apart the causes. Some patients had been seriously ill, and they typically had measurable damage to organs such as the heart or lung. The extent of the damage COVID-19 had done to them was highly unusual for a respiratory virus—and deeply alarming. But, Chen told me, "those were actually the luckier patients, because we could target treatment toward that." The unlucky remainder—more than 90 percent of the patients the center has seen—was a puzzling group "where we couldn't see what was wrong," Chen said. They were overwhelmingly women, even though men are typically hit harder by acute COVID-19. ("Acute COVID-19" refers to the distinct period of infection during which the immune system fights off the virus; the acute phase can range from mild to severe.) And they tended to be young, between the ages of twenty and fifty—not an age group that, doctors had thought, suffered the worst effects of the disease. Most of the patients were white and relatively well-off, raising concern among clinicians that many people of color might have the same ongoing symptoms but not be getting the care they needed.

In ways that will be familiar by now to readers, the long-COVID patients' tests usually showed nothing obviously the matter with them. "Everything was coming back negative," says Dayna McCarthy, a rehabilitation-medicine physician and a lead clinician at the center. "So of course Western medicine wants to say, 'You're fine.'"

But the patients were self-evidently not fine, just as I had not been fine. A survey by Patient-Led Research Collaborative for COVID-19, one of various groups drawing attention to persisting problems, asked nearly 3,800 patients with ongoing illness to describe their symptoms. A significant number—85.9 percent—reported having relapses in the months after their initial infection, usually triggered by mental or physical exertion. Many patients were experiencing severe fatigue and brain fog. Other patients suffered from chest tightness and tachycardia—a condition in which the heart beats more than a hundred times a minute—when they stood up or walked. Patient groups of COVID-19 long haulers were springing up on Facebook and elsewhere online, where people shared data and compared notes. In the spring of 2020, I began lurking on these message boards, horrified to be watching in real time as thousands of formerly healthy young people became seriously sick with chronic symptoms that were eerily familiar to me.

Early on, many doctors, predictably, dismissed these cases as the result of anxiety or hypochondria. But at Mount Sinai, Chen and other colleagues, including David Putrino, tried to figure out what was happening. Their interest was not just academic. Beyond the terrifying impact on individual lives, the scope of the problem alarmed them. "My goodness, the economic implications of this," McCarthy told me. "You're talking a huge number of twenty-to-forty-year-olds—our workforce—who now can't work." Informal estimates suggest that 10 to 30 percent of those infected with the novel coronavirus have long-term symptoms. Even if that number proves to be a massive overestimate, the number of long-COVID patients will be startlingly large. "What people need to know is the pandemic's toll is likely much higher than we are imagining," Craig Spencer, the director of global health in emergency medicine at NewYork-Presbyterian/Columbia University Irving Medical Center, told me. "It is an area that merits urgent attention. There will be people living with the impact of COVID long after the pandemic is over. This is not made up or in the minds of people who are sickly. This is real."

Based on preliminary evidence, some theories speculate that long COVID is a result of a powerful immune reaction unleashed by the virus, leaving widespread damage in the body; others posit that the immune response to the virus triggers autoimmune disease; and still other theories suggest that the virus itself causes hard-to-observe damage in the nervous system and other parts of the body, or that it remains in reservoirs hidden in the body, triggering an ongoing immune response. Or perhaps a combination of these factors is at play in different patients. (Interestingly, a significant group of patients reported that getting vaccinated resolved their symptoms.)

"What we're seeing is an entirely distinct syndrome," David Putrino told me, one that tends to be "way more debilitating and severe" than others like it, but similarly mysterious. It has become clear that many patients live with what Putrino identified as dysautonomia. Even so, the patients' symptoms were too varied to be lumped under an established label. In some ways the condition resembled dysautonomia, and POTS in particular—but it was not textbook. (Some clinicians began calling it post-COVID POTS.) In other ways, it closely resembled ME/CFS, in which people *also* demonstrate exercise intolerance and profound fatigue, but it was likewise not textbook. Same for autoimmune disorders. A commonality stood out as I interviewed researchers who described their findings: these are all poorly understood conditions that can be triggered by the body's response to infections, with clusters of system-roaming symptoms that get grouped under one name.

By chance, Putrino had been working on a project for dysautonomia patients with Amy Kontorovich, a genetic cardiologist at Mount Sinai who studies the condition and has treated hundreds of patients with it. (After they met, Kontorovich ended up diagnosing and treating Putrino's wife, who has a form of Ehlers-Danlos syndrome.) And so, as the team showed him the cases, Putrino told me, he felt a leap of recognition. "I looked at the symptoms and was like, 'Oh my god.' And I called Amy and said, 'Help.'" Kontorovich recalls that as she learned about long COVID, she had a sinking feeling. "If this is something that happens to a lot of people, we're in trouble," she remembers thinking, "because most doctors don't recognize dysautonomia as a real entity."

IF THERE IS ANY REASON for hope in the growing epidemic of long COVID, it is that some academic medical centers are taking these patients seriously. After all, medicine's history with hard-to-identify chronic illnesses, particularly those that mainly affect women, has not been good. This time, though, patient activist groups working to legitimize their suffering have met with more openness from the academic medical establishment. The NIH and the World Health Organization publicly recognized long COVID as a syndrome that warrants more research. Why are things changing? One reason is the sheer breadth of the problem. The world's attention is on COVID and its aftereffects in ways that it never was on Lyme disease or ME/CFS. But it is also because when patient groups began calling attention to long COVID, they were reaching out to clinicians who were primed to listen: many of those who first reported the experience of relapses and persistent symptoms were doctors and clinicians, including Dayna McCarthy, who struggles with long COVID. "These are doctors that we work alongside," Chen told me. "And we know that these aren't patients that are faking it. If my fellow doctor, whom I work with closely, is telling me that they can't get through the day because they can't think straight, I'm going to believe that."

In these places, too, the people treating long haulers were already champions of thinking in new ways about chronic illness. Amy Kontorovich, for instance, has been treating dysautonomia patients for almost a decade and had become passionate about advocating for those whose conditions are dismissed. "Most of my patients were young women between the ages of twenty and forty-five. And the story was often one of a long diagnostic journey," Kontorovich told me. "Patients had been told symptoms were in their head or purely due to anxiety." Her patients epitomize those the medical system frequently fails—by contesting the reality of their illness, sending them from specialist to specialist, loading them up with drugs without getting to the root cause, in all the ways we have already seen.

In places where hospital leaders are listening to such doctors, though, there is a new kind of openness to treating such patients. At Mount Sinai, for instance, when patients remained sick, rather than dismiss them Putrino's team realized that a key piece of the puzzle of long COVID was right in front of them: dysfunctional breathing. Evidence began to accrue that long-COVID patients were breathing shallowly through their mouths and into their upper chest instead of through their noses and deep into the diaphragm, which stimulates the vagus nerve that helps regulate heart rate and the autonomic nervous system. In these cases, though, the patients' breathing "is just completely off," McCarthy told me. Chen's and Putrino's teams introduced a weeklong pilot of a science-based breathwork program, designed by a company called Stasis, to try to restore normal breathing patterns in the sickest patients. After a week, everyone in the pilot program reported improvement in symptoms like shortness of breath and fatigue. It was hardly the end of their problems, but it was a clue, a start—and a sign that science could help, were it applied to their plight.

In 2012, when I got acutely sick, the idea that a major medical institution might swiftly see the need for an organized approach to persistent post-acute viral symptoms and pivot to action would have seemed beyond belief. In 2020, it happened—and not just at Mount Sinai but at other academic medical centers across the country. The dimensional, time-intensive approach Mount Sinai has taken—informed by integrative medicine, with the stated goal of "treating the whole person, not just the disease"—gives patients the best chance possible of eventually making a full, or at least fuller, recovery.

Medicine's prompt attention to long-COVID patients has mattered because successful management of the condition, whatever its specific catalyst, seems to be tied to timely treatment of it. As Putrino told me, "What we know from these sorts of conditions is the longer that you persist with the symptoms without having them managed, the longer it takes to eventually rehabilitate them." People who were seen right away tended to recover more quickly. I spoke with one patient, Caitlin Barber, who had lived for nine months with long COVID when she finally got into the Mount Sinai center in mid-September 2020—having learned about it from a patient Facebook group. When I first spoke with her, her dysautonomia was so bad that she was unable to go up and down the stairs to her apartment and was mostly bedridden. She suffered from profound brain fog—she was no longer able to work—and when she stood up, her heart raced to 180 beats per minute. (A typical heart rate is 60 to 100.) "I had been dismissed and turned down and completely gaslighted by doctors for months," she recalled. During that time, she got sicker and sicker. At the center, where Barber saw an intake doctor and was given a full cardiac evaluation, the doctors told her they believed her, and they could help, though they didn't yet know what the path toward recovery might look like. They set up coordinated appointments for her and introduced her to breathwork and gentle PT, validating her symptoms and listening to her concerns. Over time, as she followed Mount Sinai's program, Barber's symptoms improved enough that she could walk up and down the stairs; one thing that kept her going, she told me, was that now she had a *plan.*

THE WAY CAITLIN BARBER WAS treated at Mount Sinai is a model for the care of patients not only with long COVID but the kind of conditions described in this book. With Chen's sense of organizational urgency and Putrino's unconventional approaches, the Mount Sinai system, like AHN, has built a model for what more institutions can and should do for patients with chronic systemic conditions. If only there were more centers for the care of autoimmune disease, PTLDS, ME/CFS, and long COVID that helped patients get to root causes and treated common co-morbidities. These centers could be, like AHN is, set up both to research and treat the multiple overlapping factors that often accompany these illnesses.

Such care matters, because, as we've seen, access and empathy impact chronically ill patients. Caitlin Barber's coordinated day of appointments was nothing like the bare-bones ten-minute appointments that many of us are used to having with specialists who don't speak with one another. In many places in the country, such high-level medical care is hard to come by. Historically, underserved communities—whether their members are primarily rural, low income, or people of color—have had less access to such care. (Comprehensive statistics on long COVID's impact on different ethnic and socioeconomic groups have yet to be gathered.)

All of this raises the question of how—or if—we will have the resources to treat everyone in need. Hospitals make money by getting more patients in the door and out again. The care that these kinds of chronic illness demand may not be high-tech, but it is time-consuming and attention intensive. Clinicians need to tailor care to patients in ways that "our health care system is not set up for," as Dayna McCarthy put it. (This is one of the reasons that Mount Sinai's wait list has ballooned.) Medicine is used to the quick fix. This kind of syndrome, which can't be treated with a pill and stubbornly resists straightforward solutions, "is not one that doctors like treating," I heard from another doctor. As Putrino told me, many of Mount Sinai's post-acute COVID patients are "on a road to recovery. But I would not say a single one of our patients feels like they did before they got sick."

Maybe this time reform will happen, since the pandemic has delivered an unprecedented jolt to a generation of doctors and researchers. Jessica Cohen, a doctor patient who now lives with dysautonomia triggered by COVID, told me she was shocked to realize how little she'd been taught about dysautonomia in med school, given how common it really is. Getting sick has changed how she approaches caring for chronically ill patients. Meanwhile, the clock is ticking for patients whose illnesses continue to defy tidy categorization and treatment. The hurdles are profound. "A lot of clinicians want the algorithm," Putrino said. "There is no algorithm. There is listening to your patient, identifying symptoms, finding a way to measure the severity of the symptoms, applying interventions to them, and then seeing if those symptoms resolve. That is the way that medicine should be." In the meantime, the human toll expands, for all of us who live with such conditions.

TWENTY

The Wisdom
Narrative

The stories that we tell about illness are almost entirely about overcoming it, but for illnesses that cannot be overcome, they are about
growing wiser as a result of suffering. During my illness, I kept finding
that others wanted to assuage my pain by reassuring me of the good
things it had brought with it. They had embraced the reassurances
of a cultural narrative in which the ravages of illness are offset by the
enlightening spiritual knowledge they bring with them—a narrative
in which sickness is bearable because it transforms the sufferer. One
spring when I was at my most ill, a friend visited me at my apartment in
Brooklyn and, drinking herbal tea beside me on the couch where I spent
most of my days, earnestly brought up all the things my illness had
taught me. Surely, she said, such lessons were worthwhile. I bridled,
then snapped, "I would prefer not to have learned any of them this way,
to be honest."

In the American pop spiritual approach, illness is a vehicle for self-
improvement and hard-won acceptance, a line of thinking the sick patient quickly finds everywhere. It shows up in *Alice in Bed*, Susan

Sontag's play about the chronically ill Alice James. At one point, a friend blithely encourages Alice, who is at that moment extremely sick, to "want what you are capable of" and shrug off the rest. "Life is not just a question of courage," Alice tartly replies. In *The Illness Narratives*, the anthropologist Arthur Kleinman praises patients who are able to handle their illness with "grace." Onlookers often respond to the experience of chronically ill people by focusing on the supposed positives, presumably because it makes the pain of witness bearable. And of course the notion of illness as a vehicle for spiritual change has its roots in a Judeo-Christian tradition that emphasizes the instructive, even sacramental, value of human pain.

It is true that illness is an experience that tests you and forces you to rebuild your life. The destruction it wreaks makes room for re-creation. As Arthur Frank puts it in *The Wounded Storyteller*, "Unmaking can be a generative process; what is unmade stands to be remade." But I had read too many letters and diaries written by suffering people to feel sanguine about healthy friends focusing on the "spiritual growth" illness brings with it. There is a razor-thin line between trying to find something usefully redemptive in illness and lying to ourselves about the nature of suffering. Until we mourn what is lost in illness—and until we have a medical community that takes seriously the suffering of patients—we should not celebrate what is gained in it.

At various points (when I was most ill, and as I began to recover), I wrestled with whether anything good could be said to come out of chronic illness: Does illness bring wisdom? What does it mean to suffer? To answer that we need to understand in a deep way the types of stories we tell ourselves about illness—and to accept that the meaning of any given illness is unstable, indeterminate, and different from person to person.

I got sick, I got worse, I got better—that's how the standard illness narrative goes. But just as I am unable to pinpoint exactly how or when my illness started, I cannot say that it ended. My narrative is not a neat one. Which version of the story of my illness I tell depends on what month, what day, even what hour I do so, and whether my symptoms are in the background or the foreground. I am luckier than I thought I would be when I got acutely sick in 2012. After years of suffering, being treated for a tick-borne illness got me partly better, transforming me from a bed-ridden person who could not recall basic words like "spring" to a functioning and often energetic thirty-eight-year-old. I have recovered, and yet—though I try not to focus on it—I am still sick. I live with hypermobile Ehlers-Danlos syndrome, POTS, and autoimmune thyroiditis. I have on-going fatigue, brain fog, and neurological and connective tissue problems. They are mostly manageable. Sometimes they are not.

One recent morning, I woke feeling unwell. Sharp electric shocks ran along my legs and arms. I stood by the sink unable to do the dishes, twitching in pain. My older son looked up from eating his breakfast and said, "What's wrong, Mommy?" At four, he has already learned that sometimes I am unwell, despite my best efforts to hide it. It hurts me that he worries for me.

It is difficult to look at the shadows of physical suffering clearly, because to do so, I know, is to risk inviting depression, or a terrifying apprehension that the world is made of pain. But when I was at my sickest, I resolved that if I got well enough to write about my experience, I would not give false assurances. I would not write letters reassuring those I loved that my life had not been utterly compromised. Now that I am somewhat better, I can tell you the truth: When I was at my sickest, my life *was* utterly compromised, and my very sense of self was gone. When I was less sick—and there were periods of relief in my illness—I could step back from the experience and take pleasure in the vividness of the blue sky from my bedroom window. But I will not repeat falsehoods; I will not say the wisdom and growth mean I wouldn't have it any other way. I *would* have it the other way.

. . .

WHEN YOU GET SERIOUSLY ILL, either with a chronic illness or a grave disease like cancer, your sense of story is disrupted. As Arthur Frank puts it, "The body sets in motion the need for new stories when its disease disrupts the old stories," forcing the patient to "learn 'to think differently.'" The new stories we tell matter, Frank argues, because they "*repair* the damage" that being sick has done to the ill person's self-understanding.

Frank identifies three kinds of illness stories: restitution narratives, chaos narratives, and quest narratives. In restitution narratives, the sickness is bearable because the ill people believe that in the end *they will get better*. Restitution narratives emphasize recovery over the reality of illness. In fact, the restitution narrative could be called the dominant mode of late-capitalist illness narratives. As Frank notes, "Contemporary culture treats health as the normal condition that people ought to have restored." Frank himself had cancer. During his treatment, he noticed that health care workers interpreted his experiences "within a narrative of movement toward recovery of health."

Chronic illness, though, is hard to map onto a restitution narrative. It is almost by definition never a story of overcoming, because the disease's trajectory never fully resolves. And so many sick people find themselves in Frank's second kind of story, the chaos narrative. As Frank notes, "events are told as the storyteller experiences life: without sequence or discernable causality." While the idea of restitution is inherently narrative (*First I got sick, then I got better*), chaos is "anti-narrative"; these stories are hard to hear. Buffeted by endless medical tests, searching for answers, sick people are often a "narrative wreck," in a phrase Frank borrows from the legal philosopher Ronald Dworkin.

The final story is what Frank calls the quest narrative, a story in which the patient has been able to synthesize her experience into a meaning of some kind—although it's usually not the meaning (recovery) that she thought she'd find when she first got sick. Inherent in the quest narrative is "searching for alternative ways of being ill." The quest becomes clear only after the sick person experiences a deeper initiation into the world of illness, identifying the way that she has been transformed by it. In quest narratives, speakers find that the *act* of telling restores some of the control and sense of meaning they had lost. Think of Friedrich Nietzsche, who suffered from debilitating headaches, writing, "I have given a name to my pain, and call it 'dog.' . . . I can scold it and vent my bad mood on it, as others do with their dogs, servants, and wives."

The more I talked to sick people, the more I found that what is most disturbing for many of us is that grace has become a kind of moral requirement in sickness: *If you must be ill, at least be* improved *by your illness.* And yet the conditions under which grace can emerge may not be present. For one thing, it's nearly impossible to adjust to your new identity when the medical community itself refuses to recognize the physical reality of your disease—when you have no name for what ails you, or you are told it's psychosomatic. Then, too, the United States does not treat health care as a human right or sick people with dignity. How can you achieve grace if you are losing the job on which you and your children rely? Or when you feel you are materially failing those who love you?

The narrative of recovery against all odds has a powerful grip on us. In *Being Mortal,* Atul Gawande notes that the "battle of being mortal is the battle to maintain the integrity of one's life—to avoid becoming so diminished . . . that who you are becomes disconnected from who you were or who you want to be."

But one doesn't avoid this. I did not remain myself. Instead, I experienced diminishment: the tunnel I never wanted to enter, the culvert that terrified me, the threat I thought I couldn't survive. "It's bearable, and yet *I cannot bear it,*" wrote Alphonse Daudet of living with syphilis. I had revised his line in my head: "It is unbearable—*and yet I bear it.*"

I survived, but it was the nature of the disease to rob me of myself. Frank's insights into our contemporary hunger for framing illness as a kind of quest reminded me of a passage from an essay on virtue by the philosopher Alasdair MacIntyre. It makes a simple point: what the quester thinks a quest is for is never what the quest is for. A traditional medieval quest, MacIntyre argues, is not "a search for something already adequately characterized, as miners search for gold or geologists for oil." Rather, it is through "encountering and coping with the various particular harms, dangers, temptations and distractions" that "the goal of the quest is finally to be understood." The quest "is always an education . . . in self-knowledge." It entails a journey that forces the quester to be present in ways he or she might prefer not to be, and it does not necessarily involve triumph—although some part of me had always thought it did. Rather, it involves discovery. The quest turns the quester from a bad reader of circumstance, prone to sentimental expectations, to a good reader, alert to life's unseen dimensions. If the object of your illness quest is simply to get better, you are not yet deep on your quest.

As a child, lying on the couch in the summer cabin we visited, I used to read and reread the tales of King Arthur's Round Table. I remember losing myself in a place where fantasy was alive and the shadows in the room felt like doorways into great adventures. Toward the end of the tales, Galahad, who has been prophesied to be the greatest knight of all, goes on a search for the Holy Grail. Although Galahad discovers the Grail, he elects to die while still pure of soul instead of bringing it back to Camelot, where he would become a creature of worldly concerns again. The goal of his quest has shifted from returning home to achieving spiritual transformation. As a child reading this for the first time, I was saddened by Galahad's decision. The children's books I'd read had led me to believe that the heroes always came back. When I reread the tales of King Arthur, I used to stop before I got to Galahad's discovery and imagine different outcomes.

In retrospect I see that I was a bad reader from the start, in search of the easy ending, the solution. I read for what allowed me escape. I looked away from the bruises blooming in the body. I kept going back to the false goal of the quest.

As a sick person, I did not have that option. I had to become a new kind of reader. And as this reader I must acknowledge that not all stories are quests. For some people being ill remains so awful and so taxing that it brings nothing other than chaos. Perhaps coming to grasp *this* fact is the wisdom that illness brings with it.

The more I thought about it, the more I saw that the wisdom narrative was the product of some complexities worth unpacking. First, it relieved the interlocutor of feelings of anxiety about illness. If illness could be said to bring growth with it, well, then, it wasn't exactly the thing that she or he feared—it wasn't a tragedy, it wasn't a kind of prison. Instead, it was dynamic, like running a marathon or doing a wellness cleanse: a challenge, punctuated by suffering, but ultimately worth it. Second, in an era when so many of us feel busy unto death, when the culture seems to be increasingly shallow, the questions I kept getting about illness betrayed— could it be?—a kind of yearning for a forced spiritual encounter, a slowing down and reckoning that we don't find in our lives otherwise. Listening to the questions that came at me, I recognized that what my interlocutors wanted was for me to bring a spiritual flavor and framework to illness, to be to disease what Marie Kondo is to clutter. They wanted their own possible future illness to offer a necessarily radical intervention, something they might benefit from, without which they would meander along until one day they, too, were forced to confront the deeper realities of our time here. There is a reason, as the historian Jennifer Ratner-Rosenhagen has put it, that "wisdom-talk is big business in America"; in the absence of a coherent spiritual tradition, a debased popular-wisdom culture springs up in its place. Think kabbalah strings, meditation apps, positive thinking, or the trendy embrace of autoimmunity as a manifestation of the perils of modern life, for which, of course, a pricey turmeric latte powder is prescribed. (A powder I myself bought and still use.)

One might think that this appetite for news of illness-inspired growth is just what American society needs to crack open a deeper conversation about illness, a space where ill health can finally find a voice. But there's an irony here. This wisdom the ill person has gleaned is, in the first place, the result of a quest to discover why it is so problematic to be sick in this culture. From this perspective, my friend's desire to skip straight to the positive aspect of illness was itself an example of the distortion I was trying to write about: it reflected the fact that our culture tries to short-circuit the quest in order to get to the *goal*. It is, of course, an understandable impulse. I used to have it, too. "One of our most difficult duties as human beings is to listen to the voices of those who suffer," Frank writes, adding, "These voices bespeak conditions of embodiment that most of us would rather forget our own vulnerability to. Listening is hard, but it is also a fundamental moral act."

That illness does change you—this is certain.

The word "wisdom" comes from the Old English words *wis* (knowledge, learning) and *doom* (judgment). Perhaps ill people do, in a sense, become wise through encountering doom, and as a result they become new versions of themselves, having made it through some of the hazards of the course, experiencing what the poet John Ashbery calls "the charity of the hard moments." Those encounters perhaps allow us to see ourselves—and our mortal condition—more clearly.

But it would be false not to observe that this knowledge is born of loss, of resignation to a condition that forces us to give up on aspects of ourselves we had hoped we might develop. Wisdom, in this understanding, is knowledge coupled with the wound that comes from encountering doom.

BEING ILL IS A SOCIAL EXPERIENCE, as John Donne realized. It is what Frank calls "dyadic": impossible to understand without thinking about the self in relation to others. Yet Western medical culture insists on the solitariness of illness: everything about it intensifies the monadic aspect, confining patients to hospitals where anonymity differentiates and isolates rather than embraces and unifies us in our interconnected humanity. The patient's identity is thwarted, silenced, distorted in a culture that does not recognize itself in its sick members. One of the most important discoveries I made in the process of being ill is that solitary striving, my American habit of self-focus, was in some fundamental way a degradation of the most powerful aspects of our lives, which now seem to me to be our interconnectedness and need of others. I look at my small sons, and I see that they need me, and in that I see what is most meaningful in the end—not children, specifically, but the bonds among us.

I wrote all this while staying in Massachusetts, at the end of a late winter snowstorm that would make the week the snowiest in New England history. In the vast quiet, small sounds stood out, announcing themselves as the record of an already vanishing present. A black ice coated the sidewalks. In the afternoon, men dressed in puffy white coats resembling hazmat suits shoveled the snow and walked aimlessly among the drifts, futilely pushing against the whiteout that would soon cover even the parking meters. I found myself thinking of James Joyce's story "The Dead," which ends with a languorous vision of a world covered by snow: "He watched sleepily the flakes, silver and dark, falling obliquely against the lamplight. . . . His soul swooned slowly as he heard the snow falling faintly through the universe and faintly falling, like the descent of their last end, upon all the living and the dead."

The lintels of the windows were dusted in white, the whole world quiet except for the thrum of snowplows, the *beep-beep* of trucks backing up, the sounds of our present lives. I slipped into a deep calm, thinking of the living and the dead intertwined, all together beneath the flakes and the dirt of the world. It was a painful calm: a sense of how little control we have over the course of our lives and an understanding that the deepest meanings come from our contact with that portal between control and submission. This was not necessarily an expansive vision, but in its accuracy, it was, for the moment, soothing. As the poet Audre Lorde put it, of living with breast cancer, "My visions of a future I can create have been honed by the lessons of my limitations."

But I was also aware that I felt this way largely because I was not as sick as I had been. When I was at my sickest, there was little room for understanding, only for discomfort.

My illness changed me, and as a result I know more about embodiment than I used to. And some part of me is proud of that knowledge, which I raise to my lips like a bitter seed now and then, just to remember how it truly is, what this life really is about behind the façade of daily pretense, new cars, school sing-alongs, seasonal decorations, emails piling up unanswered, bills to pay, and the sweet hugs of my children with their plump limbs and fluffy snowsuits.

DURING A TRIP TO DEATH VALLEY in 2013, Jim and I had driven down to the salt flats in Badwater Basin. It was already late in the morning and the sun was high overhead. The flats stretched shockingly out before us—a vast cracked expanse of salt crystals covering a mud basin, the surface of the earth blanched a glaring white. It was so hot the heat seemed to pound at your skin, pulsing in waves. There was a path out to a vantage point, and we walked along it. The glare below and the sun above baked our skin. I got dizzy as soon as I got out of the car but focused on the signpost. Growing dizzier and dizzier, with chills flushing me, I began to feel I would never make it there, that I was living, suddenly, in Zeno's paradox. What was only a few short steps felt like miles. My limbs were watery, and my palpitating heart went liquid, as if it might leak into my body, turning me from person to lake.

At my sickest it seemed to me that my illness would never abate— that every day would be a purgatory of suffering in which my main task was merely to survive. That it did abate now feels natural to me. And so

I can tell the story of walking the salt flats without the embodied panic I felt then.

But as Audre Lorde said, "I would lie if I did not also speak of loss."

To be chronically ill is to be in a state of ever-present "camouflaged grieving," as the historian Jennifer Stitt puts it. It was this ever-present grief I felt was being swept under the rug when my friend counseled me to see the good that had come of my illness. She wasn't wrong that something had come of it—but her quick counsel negated the complexity of the quest.

Even the ill get it wrong, falsifying their experience to make it more palatable to others. In 1886, six years before her death, Alice James wrote to her friend Fanny Morse the following reassurances: "Pray dearest Fanny don't think of me as a forlorn failure but as a happy individual who has infinitely more in her life than she deserves. You know that ill or well one is never deprived of the power of standing for what one was meant to stand for & what more can life give us?" Of this passage, the critic Ruth Yeazell bluntly notes, "Even as a mere formula of consolation, this is remarkably empty." The "power of standing for what one was meant to stand for," after all, is as Yeazell notes "a purely rhetorical force, an energy whose ends are wholly undefined."

To the extent that illness is a quest, it brings you to a very different place from the one you thought you were trying to get to. And so I am wary of papering over illness's real ravages with false pieties that allow us to look away from the true price exacted.

Is illness, in any way, a lesson? Illness is a travesty; illness is shit; illness is not redemptive unless it happens to be for a particular ill person, for reasons that are not replicable nor should they be said to be so. (They usually stem from the sufferer's having reached a place in the illness that makes it more bearable than it once was.) In the dark room where I listened to life happen around me when I was sick, I yielded a part of myself forever.

This was an important event, and it is one that keeps on happening in my life. It moves in spiral time around the linear life I sometimes think I live.

As soon as I started to feel a little better, grief rushed in. Only now, some years out, having had my two sons—watching them grow in good health—does the sorrow fully flood me. I feel a black hole for what I lost: nearly the entire decade of my thirties, which might otherwise have been the best decade of my life. So many possibilities and freedoms. And why? The pain and anger are still there, inside me: flashes of the old sense that I was—or am—gradually leaving my life before I wanted to.

What I learned cannot be summarized or turned into a useful truism. It rather resembles a glint in the earth, a bit of mica on the rock that catches the sun just so. I'm always trying to turn to that sun, to be adrift in the snow-shine, to find the aspect that stuns me into a reverence I know I can't control. I will not say that this is the gift of illness, because I do not think illness is a gift. It is not anything so tangible and fixed. But this may be illness's reality, its weather, the way swaying underfoot is a quality of sea travel one only knows in full by stepping back, once more, on firm land.

I know that people reading this book might wish for a conclusion. Indeed, if I had never gotten sick, I would want, even expect, the story to crest to an uplifting finale.

But I cannot reassure any of us in the way we want. I cannot tell you that it was the green juices or the antibiotics that made me better. I don't know for sure that I had Lyme disease (though I think I did) or whether the *B. burgdorferi* bacteria are still in my body, causing the cycles of neurological symptoms that lead me to take antibiotics once again. I don't know how much my doctor's recent conclusion that I have hypermobile Ehlers-Danlos syndrome is responsible for my ongoing symptoms; it is associated with dysautonomia, pain, and fatigue. I may never learn whether—as I suspect—the collision between pathogens that seek out connective tissue and the central nervous system and my particular genetics is what led me to become extremely sick. As much as I still crave that panel on my arm that would read out exactly what was wrong at any given time, I know there is a lot I will never know. All I know is that how I ask and answer these questions has changed. And imagining that I might never have found the antibiotic treatment that has saved my life in every sense—restoring its joy—terrifies me.

I think often about patients who are less fortunate, whose disease, whatever it may be, has gone unrecognized by our medical system. One of the bitterest aspects of my illness has been this: not only did I suffer from a disease, but I suffered at the hands of a medical establishment that, for too long, failed to fully credit my testimony. The U.S. medical system not only failed to diagnose me; it stopped my quest in its tracks. Instead of acknowledging what was wrong with me, the medical system asked my body to behave as the obedient container of a distinctive and previously understood disease rather than as the site of a complex illness it didn't understand. In the throes of illness, cut off from the life you once lived, fearing that your future has been filched, what do you have but the act of witness? *This is what it is like. Please listen, so that one day you might be able to help.*

WHILE I WAS MOST ILL, I began to think about the fact that wisdom is not a goal but a process. As a process, it can always break down. I would contend that it *does* break down as soon as doctors stop recognizing the reality of a patient's illness, or dismiss the patient's pain. It can also break down when the suffering recurs without explanation. My own illness's meaning, in other words, derives also from all the ways it was *not* allowed to mean until I wrote this account of its meanings. At the start of this book, I looked at the rash on my arm and wondered what it meant. I had no way of understanding at the time everything that it would come to mean, or that its meaning lay in the complex immunological processes that led to its manifestation and to all the thoughts I would have in the years following its appearance. Its fate was mine, and my fate was its, and the "I" and the "it" had a far different relationship, I would come to know, from anything I had been capable of conceiving.

To become chronically ill is not only to have a disease that you have to manage, but to have a new story about yourself, a story that many people refuse to hear—because it is deeply unsatisfying, full of fits and starts, anger, resentment, chasms of unruly need. My own illness story has no destination. Rather, it is the sum of all of the ways it taxed and surprised me; all the people it threw me into rough contact with; all the accommodations and limitations it brought with it; the suffering I underwent; the pride I felt at times, at having endured, and at having persevered until I got a diagnosis; the years spent longing for a child before having a child. It is the fact that although I have children, those years of longing remain written on my body and etched into my soul, such as it is. The longing is with me every time I hear my younger son cry from his bed at night, or see him reach his plush, velvety, chubby arms up to me; it fills me with a guilt and overwhelming rush of love for him predicated on just how unlikely it is, to me, that he is in the world.

Sometimes I look at R, still a baby, and think I have disassociated. I am adrift in a false reality, a fantasy of escape that helps me endure. I catch myself thinking that I don't have a child, that he is part of a long dream, a deliciousness I dare not enjoy too much—or dare not stop enjoying—lest he be snatched back.

But no, I am here, in this world, facing his bright being, his young body that wants more than anything to thrive.

Inside him, his thymus is an education factory, his T cells are learning what to tag as "germ" and what to tolerate as "self." The macrophages are hungrily eating the toxins that enter through his skin, his food, his breath. Deep in the bone marrow the B cells learn.

I watch him, I put my ear against his heart and listen to the blood thrum with immunity and vulnerability.

My illness left an open window in me through which anything can climb, at any time.

ACKNOWLEDGMENTS

This book could not have been written without the assistance of grants from the Guggenheim Foundation, the Radcliffe Institute at Harvard University, and the Whiting Foundation. I am indebted to those organizations for giving me the time and space in which to think and read and start writing; special thanks to Edward Hirsch, Courtney Hodell, Sharon Bromberg-Lin, and—though she is no longer alive—Judith Vichniac for their support. Several scholars and writers with whom I was at Radcliffe became invaluable interlocutors: ZZ Packer, Jennifer Ratner-Rosenhagen, John Tasioulas, and Itai Yanai. I cannot adequately state how grateful I am for your minds; our conversations deepened this project. Harvard University generously provided me research fellows without whom this book would be far from what it is: Kaveh Danesh, Forrest Brown, Caleb Lewis, Aakriti Prasai, Eleni Apostolatos—I am grateful to this day for your hard work and all you brought to this project. Hunter Braithwaite, Michelle Ciarrocca, Isabelle Laurenzi, Sean Lynch, and Stephanie Kelley provided invaluable assistance in the fact-checking and final editing of this book, and I am extremely grateful to each of them. Susan Laity read this book early on and helped me solve many problems I hadn't been able to solve.

I am grateful to Henry Finder and David Remnick for publishing the essay from which this book grew, "What's Wrong with Me?," in *The New Yorker*; to Ann Hulbert and the team at *The Atlantic* for working with me on articles that gave rise to chapters of this book; and to Hanya Yanagihara and *T Magazine* for getting me to think about silence. Thanks to Cathy Park Hong for reading early chapters and encouraging me onward, to Jonathan Safran Foer for providing a space when I needed it, to Danielle Chapman for her wise notes, and to Deborah Landau and my colleagues in the NYU Creative Writing Program for their friendship and support. And my profound thanks to the team at *The Yale Review*, in particular Jill Hunter Pellettieri and William Frazier, for helping me carve out the time to finish this project.

James Surowiecki read this book more times than I can count and listened to me talk obsessively about this project for nearly a decade. Mary Surowiecki took care of her grandchildren many mornings so I could squeeze in a few extra hours of reading and revision. During the many weeks that I wrote this book, Sunita Jagnath and Saturnina Cooper looked after my children while I worked. This book would not exist without their labor.

I am deeply indebted to my editor, Sarah McGrath, for her patience and wisdom in guiding me through drafts, to Geoff Kloske for his support throughout, and to Delia Taylor for all her help along the way. And thank you to the entire wonderful team at Riverhead Books: I couldn't ask for a better publisher for my work. Megan Lynch had the confidence that an article could become a book, and Chris Calhoun, my agent, steadily advised me through it all.

My profound thanks are due to all the people living with chronic illness who allowed me and my team to interview them; I wasn't able to quote from each interview, but your generous input shaped how I thought about this book and what mattered most.

Finally, my current doctors and specialists epitomize the ethic of care that I call for in this book. Although this book is critical of the medical system, without their hard work and insights I would never have been able to write it. They show me the path forward.

NOTES

INTRODUCTION

3   "gradually and then suddenly": Ernest Hemingway, *The Sun Also Rises* (New York: Scribner, 2014), 109.

5   They now affect: Exact numbers are hard to come by. A report of the NIH Autoimmune Diseases Coordinating Committee titled *Progress in Autoimmune Diseases Research* (March 2005) estimates that between 14.7 million and 23.5 million Americans live with autoimmune disease. A 2012 news release from the NIH notes, "More than 32 million people in the United States have autoantibodies, which are proteins made by the immune system that target the body's tissues and define a condition known as autoimmunity, a study shows." Today, the Autoimmune Association (formerly known as the American Autoimmune Related Diseases Association) estimates, based on prevalence and population, that the number is closer to 50 million. American Autoimmune Related Diseases Association and National Coalition of Autoimmune Patient Groups, *The Cost Burden of Autoimmune Disease: The Latest Front in the War on Healthcare Spending* (2011), 2.

6   multiple sclerosis as a form of hysteria: Colin Lee Talley, "The emergence of multiple sclerosis, 1870–1950: A puzzle of historical epidemiology," *Perspectives in Biology and Medicine* 48, no. 3 (2005): 383–95.

6   a disease that afflicted: Sontag, *Illness as Metaphor*, 24–36; David S. Barnes, *The Making of a Social Disease: Tuberculosis in Nineteenth-Century France* (Berkeley: University of California Press, 1995).

7   though "chronic illness" is of course: I use "chronic illness" as a category that encompasses "poorly understood illness." I understand that there are profound differences between, say, chronic obstructive pulmonary disease (COPD) and an autoimmune disease, but I also suspect that aspects of my experience will speak to

many who live with a persistent condition, whether or not it is well understood. (To some degree, any illness is mystifying to the person who has it.) It is my hope that the lived experience described here may reveal something what it's like to live with any chronic disease. Meditating on my illness experience sometimes led me to reflect specifically on chronicity—the unendingness of it all—along with the specific issues raised by my own hard-to-diagnose condition.

CHAPTER ONE: "GRADUALLY AND THEN SUDDENLY"

12   **the way my pain had been relegated:** It took me fourteen years to be diagnosed with endometriosis, during which I suffered from health-related quality of life issues. Endometriosis is a chronic disease in which endometrial tissue that lines the uterus is found outside the uterus; it causes extreme pelvic pain and infertility in some patients. While it is not currently considered an autoimmune condition, it is a disease driven by inflammation and, evidence suggests, seems to indicate a higher risk for autoimmune diseases. See Elizabeth García-Gómez et al., "Regulation of Inflammation Pathways and Inflammasome by Sex Steroid Hormones in Endometriosis," *Frontiers in Endocrinology* 10, no. 935 (2020). The patient's experience of endometriosis offers a prime example of modern medicine's failure to treat and study women: One 2011 study found that on average, patients across ten countries experienced a 6.7-year diagnostic delay, during which they suffered from reduced quality of life and impaired ability to work. I personally found that acupuncture treatment and eliminating gluten helped manage my endometriosis. Kelechi E. Nnoaham et al., "Impact of endometriosis on quality of life and work productivity: A multicenter study across ten countries," *Fertility and Sterility* 96, no. 2 (2011): 366–73.

16   **ulcerative colitis, and thyroid conditions:** There is extensive autoimmune disease on both sides of my family. In fact, autoimmunity often clusters in families, and yet most doctors do not ask about autoimmune disease in the family history section of patient intake forms. Asking about this history might help doctors and patients recognize, or even discover, a preexisting family history that could offer clues about the possible role of autoimmune disease in a patient's symptoms. Dr. E was the first doctor I saw—of the many doctors I'd seen in my life—who asked me questions that elicited this family history.

17   **which leaves people sluggish and foggy:** "Thyroiditis" refers to inflammation of the thyroid gland, which helps control metabolism via the hormones T4 and T3. In autoimmune thyroiditis, the immune system actively attacks the thyroid itself, damaging the organ. Early in the course of the disease, inflammation can (rarely) lead to overproduction of the hormone; as the damage to the thyroid accumulates and it "burns out" it no longer produces sufficient thyroid hormone, leading the patient to swing through a confusing array of symptoms. Symptoms may include sluggishness or anxiety and sweats, as well as hair loss and feeling cold. Today, medicine tends to search for thyroid disease by measuring levels of the "thyroid-stimulating hormone" (TSH) released by your pituitary gland in response to plummeting levels of T3 and T4. (Your pituitary gland sits below your hypothalamus and regulates key parts of your endocrine system.) In my case, it turned out, my TSH looked normal because something was wrong with my pituitary, a problem that was later identified in a diagnostic test known as "TRH stimulation thyroid test." Eventually, when Dr. E did a full test of all my thyroid-related hormones, she found that my T3 and T4 were low, although my TSH looked normal.

CHAPTER TWO: WHAT IS AN AUTOIMMUNE DISEASE?

20 "self and non-self": See Warwick Anderson and Ian R. Mackay, *Intolerant Bodies: A Short History of Autoimmunity* (Baltimore: Johns Hopkins University Press, 2014), and William E. Paul, *Immunity* (Baltimore: Johns Hopkins University Press, 2015). I rely heavily on Anderson and Mackay's seminal and important work on autoimmunity throughout this book. The information in this passage is also based on interviews with Noel R. Rose, director and founder of the Johns Hopkins Center for Autoimmune Disease Research, in May 2013 and February 2015.

20 Ehrlich's theory: Arthur Silverstein, "Autoimmunity Versus Horror Autotoxicus: The Struggle for Recognition," *Nature Immunology* 2, no. 4 (May 2001): 279–81.

21 the body could, in fact: Interviews with Rose.

21 scientists have discovered: As of July 1, 2021, the Autoimmune Association website listed more than one hundred autoimmune diseases at https://www.aarda.org /diseaselist/.

22 A 2020 study found that: Gregg E. Dinse et al., "Increasing Prevalence of Antinuclear Antibodies in the United States," *Arthritis and Rheumatology* 72, no. 6 (June 2020): 1026–35.

22 including diet and its effect on the microbiome: Dinse et al., "Increasing Prevalence of Antinuclear Antibodies."

22 approximately 80 percent of autoimmune patients: Fariha Angum et al., "The Prevalence of Autoimmune Disorders in Women: A Narrative Review," *Cureus* 12, no. 5 (May 2020): e8094.

22 "represent a major disease burden": Anderson and Mackay, *Intolerant Bodies*, 1.

22 the annual cost of autoimmune diseases: American Autoimmune Related Diseases Association and National Coalition of Autoimmune Patient Groups, *The Cost Burden of Autoimmune Disease: The Latest Front in the War on Healthcare Spending* (2011), 5.

23 an average of three years: See https://medicalresearch.com/author-interviews/survey -finds-autoimmune-diseases-are-misunderstood-common-and-underfunded/44 986/. The time to reach a diagnosis for autoimmune disease appears to be improving. When I wrote about autoimmune diseases for *The New Yorker* in 2013, Virginia T. Ladd, then president of AARDA, told me that on average patients received a diagnosis of an autoimmune disease only after five years, during which they saw five doctors.

23 "The train's gone off the tracks": Interviews with Rose.

23 As it is, many clinicians assume: According to the *Oxford English Dictionary*, the term "worried well" was coined in a 1970 *Scientific American* article by a physician named Sidney Garfield, who was taxonomizing kinds of patients: "the well," "the worried well," "the early sick," and "the sick." It is interesting that "the worried well" is a term I have frequently seen in print, whereas "the early sick"—perhaps the accurate term for me in 2007—is not a term I had come across until I read Garfield's article. This discrepancy itself tells you something about our culture's appetite for ascribing subjective symptoms to the mind rather than viewing them as evidence of a not-yet-measurable or still poorly understood disease. Sidney R. Garfield, "The Delivery of Medical Care," *Scientific American* 222, no. 4 (April 1970): 15–23.

24 "It is hardly possible": Susan Sontag, *Illness as Metaphor and AIDS and Its Metaphors* (New York: Farrar, Straus and Giroux, 2003), 3.

26 one of them a doctor: Terry Wahls, *The Wahls Protocol: A Radical New Way to Treat All Chronic Autoimmune Conditions Using Paleo Principles* (New York: Avery, 2014).

28 **feel tired and achy:** The microbiome is the community of microorganisms that inhabit our intestines and bodies. Research shows that they not only help digest food but also influence gene expression. The theory is that a processed diet can lead to excess inflammation and a condition called "leaky gut," in which the usually tightly sealed walls of the intestine become inflamed and full of gaps, so that tiny molecules pass through them. Those molecules shouldn't be in the blood, the theory goes, so the immune system starts mounting attacks on them; along the way, it makes mistakes, confused by something called "molecular mimicry." Alessio Fasano, "Leaky Gut and Autoimmune Diseases," *Clinical Reviews in Allergy and Immunology* 42, no. 1 (2012): 71–78; Salvatore Benvenga and Fabrizio Guarneri, "Molecular Mimicry and Autoimmune Thyroid Disease," *Reviews in Endocrine and Metabolic Disorders* 17, no. 4 (2016): 485–98.

32 **she said agreeably:** My doctor was willing to shift gears like this because my thyroid hormones had an unusual pattern. My free T4 and free T3 were a little low, but my TSH was not high; in fact, it had gone under 1. Dr. E was highly responsive to my input.

32 **"like a dragon on":** Robert Lowell, "Waking Early Sunday Morning," in *Near the Ocean* (New York: Farrar, Straus and Giroux, 1967).

CHAPTER THREE: DISEASE CONCEPTS

35 **could lead to all kinds of problems:** Julietta A. Sheng et al., "The Hypothalamic-Pituitary-Adrenal Axis," *Frontiers in Behavioral Neuroscience* (January 13, 2021): 1–21. For more about the hypothalamic-pituitary-adrenal axis, see https://www.neuroscientificallychallenged.com/blog/2014/5/31/what-is-the-hpa-axis.

35 **key factor in unexplained exhaustion:** For example, James L. Wilson's *Adrenal Fatigue: The 21st Century Stress Syndrome* (Petaluma, CA: Smart Publications, 2001).

36 **"the Chinese doctor . . . distinguishes":** Ted Kaptchuk, *The Web That Has No Weaver: Understanding Chinese Medicine* (New York: McGraw-Hill Education, 2000), 6.

37 **"There is no simple one-dimensional way":** Warwick Anderson and Ian R. Mackay, *Intolerant Bodies: A Short History of Autoimmunity* (Baltimore: Johns Hopkins University Press, 2014), xi.

38 **"suddenly concluded that the whole art":** George Bernard Shaw, *The Doctor's Dilemma* (London: Penguin New Edition, 1987).

38 **advances in lab testing:** Charles E. Rosenberg, *Our Present Complaint: American Medicine, Then and Now* (Baltimore: Johns Hopkins University Press, 2007), loc. 47, Kindle.

38 **"no longer concerned with man":** As quoted in Anderson and Mackay, *Intolerant Bodies*, 17.

39 **A 2018 study:** J. B. Harley et al., "Transcription factors operate across disease loci, with EBNA2 implicated in autoimmunity," *Nature Genetics* 50, no. 5 (May 2018): 699–707.

39 **Researchers at Stanford and Columbia are exploring:** K. Chang, H. S. Koplewicz, and R. Steingard, "Special issue on pediatric acute-onset neuropsychiatric syndrome," *Journal of Child and Adolescent Psychopharmacology* 25, no. 1 (February 2015): 1–2. For more on the emerging science of how infections trigger mental health conditions, see Harriet A. Washington's *Infectious Madness: The Surprising Science of How We "Catch" Mental Illness* (New York: Little, Brown, 2015).

40 **the Ebola virus may linger:** Gibrilla F. Deen, Nathalie Broutet, Wenbo Xu, et al.,

"Ebola RNA Persistence in Semen of Ebola Virus Disease Survivors—Final Report," *The New England Journal of Medicine* 377, no. 15 (October 12, 2017): 1428–37.

40 **"tense tempo of modern life"**: My account of the history about ulcers is drawn largely from Terence Monmaney's "Marshall's Hunch," *The New Yorker*, September 20, 1993, 64–72, and Michael Specter's "Germs Are Us," *The New Yorker*, October 22, 2012, 32–39.

41 **the "Semmelweis reflex"**: The Semmelweis reflex—medicine's habitual rejection of paradigm-shifting ideas—is named for the obstetrician Ignaz Semmelweis, who in the mid-nineteenth century proposed that doctors themselves were causing the childbed fever that killed many women by transporting germs to them. He made his medical staff start washing their hands with chlorine before delivering babies and noticed a decline in maternal deaths. Semmelweis's idea was, as he later noted in a medical paper, "attacked" and "rejected" by colleagues, who lectured in medical schools on its fallacies. He became obsessed by the topic of childbed fever and later went mad. For more on Semmelweis, see Theodore Obenchain's *Genius Belabored: Childbed Fever and the Tragic Life of Ignaz Semmelweis* (Tuscaloosa: University of Alabama Press, 2016). A recent example of the Semmelweis reflex at work may be how long it took researchers, in the face of overwhelming evidence, to acknowledge the airborne transmission of COVID-19. See https://deepdive.tips/index.php/2021/06/21/017-airborne-transmission-and-the-semmelweis-reflex-with-dr-david-fisman/ and Zeynep Tufekci, "Why Did It Take So Long to Accept the Facts About COVID?," *The New York Times*, May 7, 2021, https://www.nytimes.com/2021/05/07/opinion/coronavirus-airborne-transmission.html.

42 **One study found that *H. pylori***: Specter, "Germs Are Us."

43 **Complicating germ theory's paradigm**: Much about this process is still poorly understood. For an overview of some of the research on when and how viruses trigger autoimmune disease, see Maria K. Smatti et al., "Viruses and Autoimmunity: A Review on the Potential Interaction and Molecular Mechanisms," *Viruses* 11, no. 8 (August 19, 2019): 762.

43 **As Charles Rosenberg notes**: Anderson and Mackay, *Intolerant Bodies*, xi.

44 **the allostatic load**: See B. S. McEwen and E. Stellar, "Stress and the Individual: Mechanisms Leading to Disease," *Archives of Internal Medicine* 153, no. 18 (September 1993): 2093–101, and B. S. McEwen, "Stress, Adaptation, and Disease: Allostasis and Allostatic Load," *Annals of the New York Academy of Sciences* 840 (May 1, 1998): 33–44.

44 **"an era in which medicine's central premise"**: Susan Sontag, *Illness as Metaphor and AIDS and Its Metaphors* (New York: Farrar, Straus and Giroux, 2003), 5.

45 **The protagonist's mentor**: Sinclair Lewis, *Arrowsmith* (New York: New American Library, 2011), 274.

CHAPTER FOUR: IMPERSONATION

47 **"Pain is always new to the sufferer"**: Alphonse Daudet, *In the Land of Pain*, trans. Julian Barnes (New York: Alfred A. Knopf, 2003).

48 **This does not mean that the illness is in the mind**: This phenomenon of the mind affecting disease has been powerfully observed in COPD, for example. See Patricia Hill Bailey, "The Dyspnea-Anxiety-Dyspnea Cycle—COPD Patients' Stories of Breathlessness: 'It's Scary / When You Can't Breathe,'" *Qualitative Health Research* 14, no. 6 (July 2004): 760–78.

48   "loss of self": Kathy Charmaz, "Loss of Self: A Fundamental Form of Suffering in the Chronically Ill," *Sociology of Health and Illness* 5, no. 2 (1983): 168–95.

49   "Farewell me, cherished me": Daudet, *In the Land of Pain*, 31.

49   "English, which can express": Virginia Woolf, *On Being Ill* (Ashfield, MA: Paris Press, 2002), 6–7.

50   "Physical pain does not simply resist": Elaine Scarry, *The Body in Pain: The Making and Unmaking of the World* (Oxford: Oxford University Press, 1987), 4.

51   "tension myositis syndrome" (TMS): See John Sarno, *Healing Back Pain: The Mind-Body Connection* (New York: Grand Central, 1991) and *The Mindbody Prescription: Healing the Body, Healing the Pain* (New York: Grand Central, 1998).

53   "Whenever you offer an account": Christina Crosby, *A Body, Undone: Living On After Great Pain* (New York: New York University Press, 2016), 19.

54   "a slight hysterical tendency": Charlotte Perkins Gilman, "The Yellow Wallpaper," in *Herland, The Yellow Wall-Paper, and Selected Writings* (New York: Penguin Books, 1999), 166.

55   "To him who waits": Alice James, *The Diary of Alice James*, ed. Leon Edel (New York: Dodd, Mead & Company, 1964), 206.

55   So challenging was living with: In addition to James's *Diary*, I relied on Jean Strouse's *Alice James: A Biography* (New York: New York Review of Books Classics, 2011) for my understanding of James's plight.

CHAPTER FIVE: THE DOCTOR-PATIENT RELATIONSHIP

58   inflammatory and autoimmune diseases can affect the brain: Matthew S. Kayser and Josep Dalmau, "The emerging link between autoimmune disorders and neuropsychiatric disease," *The Journal of Neuropsychiatry and Clinical Neurosciences* 23, no. 1 (2011): 90–97.

59   Some doctors flat-out told me: The debate over medical records being available to patients is a cost-benefit issue, ultimately. Doctors historically have not wanted patients to have records, because the information in them is often specialized and to interpret them with reasonable nuance can require technical proficiency that patients lack. In the internet era, patients googling test results without a doctor present can lead to panicked phone calls and anxious patients. But those costs, I would argue, are outweighed by the fact that it's your body, and you deserve to have all the information you can about what's gone wrong with it. Still, it would be reasonable for doctors and patients to work together toward explicit expectation setting.

59   The 21st Century Cures Act: The 21st Century Cures Act, Pub. L. No. 114-255, 533 Stat (2016).

60   "numbers on charts": Charles E. Rosenberg, *Our Present Complaint: American Medicine, Then and Now* (Baltimore: Johns Hopkins University Press, 2007), loc. 46, Kindle.

61   "Any patient in a hospital": Terrence Holt, *Internal Medicine: A Doctor's Stories* (New York: Liveright, 2014), 126.

61   can all be barriers to good care: Jay Bhatt and Priya Bathija, "Ensuring Access to Quality Health Care in Vulnerable Communities," *Academic Medicine* 93, no. 9 (2018): 1271–75.

61   Overt racism and unconscious bias: In 2014, a number of books were published testifying to the strain in the doctor and patient relationship, several of which document this type of name-calling of patients by doctors: Sandeep Jauhar's *Doctored: The Disillusionment of an American Physician* (New York: Farrar, Straus and Giroux,

2014); Barron H. Lerner's *The Good Doctor: A Father, a Son, and the Evolution of Medical Ethics* (Boston: Beacon Press, 2014); Jack Cochran and Charles C. Kenney's *The Doctor Crisis: How Physicians Can, and Must, Lead the Way to Better Health Care* (New York: Public Affairs, 2014); and Terrence Holt's *Internal Medicine.*

61 **to provide routine care to transgender patients:** National LGBTQ Task Force Survey, https://www.thetaskforce.org/new-report-reveals-rampant-discrimination -against-transgender-people-by-health-providers-high-hiv-rates-and-widespread -lack-of-access-to-necessary-care-2/; and Deirdre A. Shires, Daphna Stroumsa, Kim D. Jaffee, and Michael R. Woodford, "Primary Care Clinicians' Willingness to Care for Transgender Patients," *The Annals of Family Medicine* 16, no. 6 (November 2018): 555–558.

61 **epitomized in the decades-long Tuskegee experiment:** See, among many others, Jinbin Park, "Historical Origins of the Tuskegee Experiment: The Dilemma of Public Health in the United States," *Uisahak* 26, no. 3 (December 2017): 545–78, and Olivia B. Waxman's "How the Public Learned About the Infamous Tuskegee Syphilis Study," *Time*, July 25, 2017.

61 **No wonder many patients distrust doctors:** The Tuskegee study appears to have had a direct impact on Black men's trust in doctors in the United States; see Marcella Alsan and Marianne Wanamaker, "Tuskegee and the Health of Black Men," *The Quarterly Journal of Economics* 133, no. 1 (February 2018): 407–55.

62 **"heartsink patients":** T. C. O'Dowd, "Five Years of Heartsink Patients in General Practice," *The British Medical Journal*, 297, no. 6647 (1988): 528–30.

63 **"To speak our life as we feel it":** Deborah Levy, *The Cost of Living: An Autobiography* (New York: Bloomsbury, 2019), chapter 1, loc. 94, Kindle.

63 **after eleven seconds:** N. Singh Ospina, K. A. Phillips, R. Rodriguez-Gutierrez, et al., "Eliciting the Patient's Agenda—Secondary Analysis of Recorded Clinical Encounters," *Journal of General Internal Medicine* 34 (2019): 36–40.

63 **"the treatment of chronic disease":** Colin Campbell and Gill McGauley, "Doctor-Patient Relationships in Chronic Illness: Insights from Forensic Psychiatry," *British Medical Journal* (Clinical Research Edition) 330, no. 7492 (2005): 667–70.

64 **doctors surveyed felt inadequately trained:** Catherine Hoffman and Dorothy Rice, *Chronic Conditions: Making the Case for Ongoing Care*, The Partnership for Solutions at Johns Hopkins University and the Robert Wood Johnson Foundation, 1996; updated September 2004. Accessible online at http://www.partnershipforsolutions .org/DMS/files/chronicbook2004.pdf.

64 **"The best kind of patient for this purpose":** T. F. Main, "The Ailment," *British Journal of Medical Psychology* 30 (September 1957): 129–45.

64 **typical medical appointment is fifteen minutes:** A 2007 study analyzed visit durations and estimated that the median length of a doctor's visit is 15.7 minutes; see Ming Tai-Seale et al., "Time allocation in primary care office visits," *Health Services Research* 42, no. 5 (2007): 1871–94. For a good explanation of why doctors' appointments are so short, see https://www.kevinmd.com/blog/2014/05/10-minutes -doctor.html. The phenomenon that Steven M. Schimpff describes in the blog post is why many of the doctors I saw had stopped taking insurance.

64 **The short appointments have a history:** My understanding of the history of American health care is drawn from Paul Starr's *The Social Transformation of American Medicine: The Rise of a Sovereign Profession and the Making of a Vast Industry* (New York: Basic Books, 2017); Charles R. Rosenberg's *Our Present Complaint*; and David Cutler's *The Quality Cure: How Focusing on Health Care Quality Can Save Your Life and Lower Spending Too* (Berkeley: University of California Press, 2014).

64 **To rein in costs:** Studies estimate that today's doctors and hospitalists—medical practitioners who do most of their work in hospitals—spend just 12 to 17 percent of their day with patients. The rest of the time is devoted to processing forms, reviewing lab results, maintaining electronic medical records, and dealing with other staff. Physicians in medical practices in the United States "spend ten times as many hours on nonclinical administrative duties" as their Canadian counterparts do, Danielle Ofri reports in *What Doctors Feel: How Emotions Affect the Practice of Medicine* (Boston: Beacon Press, 2014).

65 **Silos fail to support:** Margaret F. Schulte, "Editorial," *Frontiers of Health Services Management* 29, no. 4 (Summer 2013): 1–2.

65 **"The greater one's income":** See "How Are Income and Wealth Linked to Health and Longevity?" from the Urban Institute and the Center for Society and Wealth, https://www.urban.org/sites/default/files/publication/49116/2000178-How-are -Income-and-Wealth-Linked-to-Health-and-Longevity.pdf.

65 **"Racism is a public health emergency":** *The Lancet* 395 (June 13, 2020), https:// www.thelancet.com/journals/lancet/article/PIIS0140-6736(20)31353-2/fulltext. See also https://www.thelancet.com/series/america-equity-equality-in-health.

66 **"The patient really isn't a person":** Laurie Peterson, "Live from Davos: Aetna CEO on Health, Reinvention, and Yoga," *Yahoo News*, January 22, 2014, https://news .yahoo.com/2014-01-22-live-from-davos-aetna-ceo-on-health-reinvention-and -yoga-vide.html.

67 **distancing themselves self-protectively:** Mohammadreza Hojat et al., "An Empirical Study of Decline in Empathy in Medical School," *Medical Education* 38, no. 9 (September 2004): 934–41; Daniel C. R. Chen et al., "Characterizing Changes in Student Empathy Throughout Medical School," *Medical Teaching* 34, no. 4 (2012): 305–11. See also Hojat et al., "The Devil Is in the Third Year: A Longitudinal Study of Empathy in Medical School," *Academy of Medicine* 84, no. 9 (September 2009): 1182–91.

67 **patients benefit clinically from:** Frans Derksen et al., "Effectiveness of empathy in general practice: A systematic review," *The British Journal of General Practice* 63, no. 606 (2013): e76–84; see also Stefano Del Canale et al., "The relationship between physician empathy and disease complications: An empirical study of primary care physicians and their diabetic patients in Parma, Italy," *Academic Medicine* 87, no. 9 (2012): 1243–49.

67 **the incidence of severe diabetes complications:** Ofri, *What Doctors Feel*, 57.

68 **the group treated by the empathetic researcher:** Ted J. Kaptchuk et al., "Components of placebo effect: Randomised controlled trial in patients with irritable bowel syndrome," *British Medical Journal* (Clinical Research Edition) 336, no. 7651 (2008): 999–1003.

68 **"What Kaptchuk demonstrated":** Nathanael Johnson, "Forget the Placebo Effect: It's the 'Care Effect' That Matters," *Wired*, January 18, 2013, https://www.wired .com/2013/01/dr-feel-good/.

68 **the effects of empathy are real:** The examples abound: "Comfort talk," an approach developed by a radiologist at Beth Israel Deaconess Medical Center, has been clinically shown to reduce pain in breast biopsies and other invasive procedures, reducing the need in the case of endovascular catheterizations—which remove cardiovascular blockage—for analgesics and anesthesia by 50 percent and reducing patient anxiety as well. These upsides save money and time, decreasing the duration of patients' stays in catheterization rooms by seventeen minutes and resulting in a 40 percent reduction in MRI noncompletion rate due to patient claustrophobia. (It's worth nothing that these changes save money not for hospitals but for patients and insurance

companies, which may have something to do with why doctors and hospitals have been slow to embrace these techniques.) See Elvira V. Lang et al., "Adjunctive self-hypnotic relaxation for outpatient medical procedures: A prospective randomized trial with women undergoing large core breast biopsy," *Pain* 126, nos. 1–3 (2006): 155–64.

68   **patients who received a nonsurgical "treatment":** J. Bruce Moseley et al., "A Controlled Trial of Arthroscopic Surgery for Osteoarthritis of the Knee," *The New England Journal of Medicine* 347 (July 2002): 81–88.

68   **The rise of patients' rights:** I rely on Starr and Lerner for my understanding of the history of patients' rights. For more on informed consent, see Tom L. Beauchamp, "Informed Consent: Its History, Meaning, and Present Challenges," *Cambridge Quarterly of Healthcare Ethics* 20, no. 4 (2011): 515–23.

69   **Doctors still label:** Danielle Ofri, "When the Patient Is 'Non-Compliant,'" *The New York Times*, November 15, 2012.

69   **reform such uses of language:** Neil D. Shah and Michael W. Fried, "Treatment options of patients with chronic hepatitis C who have failed prior therapy," *Clinical Liver Disease* 7, no. 2 (2016): 40–44. Medicine has committed to linguistic reform and seven years after I began writing this book it is more common to read about "treatment failure" than "patients failing therapy."

69   **"One of the most venerable":** Richard Gunderman, "Illness as Failure: Blaming Patients," *Hastings Center Report* 30, no. 4 (2000): 7–11.

71   **Dr. Francis W. Peabody instructed:** Francis W. Peabody, "The Care of the Patient," *The Journal of the American Medical Association* 88, no. 12 (1927): 877–82.

71   **the body remains "dyadic":** Arthur Frank, *The Wounded Storyteller* (Chicago: University of Chicago Press, 2013), loc. 710, Kindle. As Frank writes, "The dyadic relation is the recognition that even though the other is a body outside of mine . . . this other *has to do with me, as I with it.*"

CHAPTER SIX: ALTERNATIVES

73   **"To the extent that modern physicalist medicine":** Anne Harrington, *The Cure Within: A History of Mind-Body Medicine* (New York: W. W. Norton, 2009), 18.

74   **Americans were spending $30.2 billion a year:** See this press release for a 2016 survey by the NIH: https://www.nccih.nih.gov/news/press-releases/americans-spent -302-billion-outofpocket-on-complementary-health-approaches. See also https:// www.cdc.gov/nchs/data/nhsr/nhsr095.pdf.

74   **"What the language of alternative medicine understands":** Eula Biss, *On Immunity: An Inoculation* (Minneapolis: Graywolf Press, 2014), loc. 467, Kindle.

77   **Whether such extraction is beneficial:** Perrine Hoet, Vincent Haufroid, and Dominique Lison, "Heavy metal chelation tests: The misleading and hazardous promise," *Archives of Toxicology* 94, no. 8 (2020): 2893–896.

77   **A study of toddlers:** See the American Academy of Pediatrics website, "Treatment of Lead Poisoning": https://www.aap.org/en-us/advocacy-and-policy/aap-health-initiatives /lead-exposure/Pages/Treatment-of-Lead-Poisoning.aspx.

77   **patients over fifty treated with chelation:** Roni Caryn Rabin, "Trial of Chelation Therapy Shows Benefits, but Doubts Persist," *The New York Times*, April 15, 2013, https://well.blogs.nytimes.com/2013/04/15/trial-of-chelation-therapy-shows -benefits-but-doubts-persist/.

80   **two polymorphisms in the MTHFR gene:** A polymorphism is a DNA variant that is more common than a genetic mutation. (Medical science currently uses "mutation"

only for variants that are found in less than 1 percent of the population.) See this site for more on the MTHFR genetic polymorphisms and their implications: https://medlineplus.gov/genetics/gene/mthfr/#conditions.

CHAPTER SEVEN: DOWNWARD SPIRAL

82 **Western medicine doesn't put much stock:** Elana Lavine, "Blood testing for sensitivity, allergy or intolerance to food," *Canadian Medical Association Journal* 184, no. 6 (2012): 666–68.

82 **gluten and eggs:** Three years later I would test positive for anti-gliadin antibodies, which can be an indicator of celiac disease or non-celiac gluten sensitivity.

83 **symbolize artisanal hipster health:** Tom Philpott, "Sorry, Foodies: We're About to Ruin Kale," *Mother Jones,* July 15, 2015.

84 **As Salzberg told David Freedman:** David H. Freedman, "The Triumph of New-Age Medicine," *The Atlantic,* July-August 2011.

84 **third leading cause of death:** M. A. Makary and M. Daniel, "Medical error—the third leading cause of death in the US," *British Medical Journal* 353 (2016): i2139.

85 **kick in your parasympathetic system:** Qian-Qian Li et al., "Acupuncture effect and central autonomic regulation," *Evidence-Based Complementary and Alternative Medicine: eCAM* 2013 (2013): 267959.

97 **"I don't believe I will get better":** Alphonse Daudet, *In the Land of Pain*, trans. Julian Barnes (New York: Alfred A. Knopf, 2003), 79.

98 **"The knowledge that you're ill":** Anatole Broyard, *Intoxicated by My Illness: And Other Writings on Life and Death* (New York: New York: Fawcett, 1993), 37, 41.

98 **"added a fierce intensity to my life":** "Susan Sontag Found Crisis of Cancer Added a Fierce Intensity to Life," *The New York Times,* January 30, 1978, https://archive.nytimes.com/www.nytimes.com/books/00/03/12/specials/sontag-cancer.html.

98 **"that little shiver of pleasure-horror":** Christian Wiman, *He Held Radical Light: The Art of Faith, the Faith of Art* (New York: Farrar, Straus and Giroux, 2018), 11.

99 **"Who would have thought my shriveled heart":** George Herbert, "The Flower," in *The Poetical Works of George Herbert* (New York: George Bell and Sons, 1886). Available on the Poetry Foundation website at https://www.poetryfoundation.org/poems/50700/the-flower-56d22df9112c4.

CHAPTER EIGHT: THE WOMAN PROBLEM

103 **One of the punitive fantasies:** Susan Sontag, *Conversations with Susan Sontag*, ed. Leland Poague (Jackson: University Press of Mississippi, 1997), 197.

103 **The stereotype of the sickly woman:** Interview with Amy Proal, May 2021.

103 **"have been labeled hypochondriacs":** From the American Autoimmune Related Diseases Association newsletter *InFocus,* 22, no. 1 (March 2014), https://www.aarda.org/wp-content/uploads/2017/02/InFocus-03-2014.pdf.

103 **nothing physical was wrong with them:** Most of the women I interviewed were cisgender; the doubt they faced from doctors underscores how even those who identify with their given sex encounter disbelief from clinicians. Evidence shows that this problem is further compounded for transgender and non-binary patients, whose relationships to their bodies do not fit neatly into the often-outdated normative frameworks that medicine relies on.

105 **Medicine treats women differently:** Barbara Ehrenreich and Deirdre English, *For Her Own Good: Two Centuries of the Experts' Advice to Women* (New York: Anchor Books, 2005). Ehrenreich and English's work, as well as Charles Rosenberg and

Carroll Smith-Rosenberg's, was a starting point for much of my understanding of the history of medicine's approach to women.

105 **Researchers do not include female mice:** Roni Caryn Rabin, "Health Researchers Will Get $10.1 Million to Counter Gender Bias in Studies," *The New York Times*, September 23, 2014, https://www.nytimes.com/2014/09/23/health/23gender.html.

105 **historically underrepresented in clinical studies of beta-blockers:** Raffaele Bugiardini et al., "Prior Beta-Blocker Therapy for Hypertension and Sex-Based Differences in Heart Failure Among Patients with Incident Coronary Heart Disease," *Hypertension* 76, no. 3 (2020): 819–26, https://doi.org/10.1161/HYPERTENSIONAHA.120.15323.

106 **"It matters":** Institute of Medicine (U.S.) Committee on Understanding the Biology of Sex and Gender Differences, *Exploring the Biological Contributions to Human Health: Does Sex Matter?*, ed. T. M. Wizemann and M. L. Pardue (Washington, DC: National Academies Press, 2001), x. Available from https://www.ncbi.nlm.nih.gov/books/NBK222288/.

106 **"We literally know less":** Rabin, "Health Researchers Will Get $10.1 Million."

106 **One such drug is Ambien:** See the official website of U.S. Food and Drug Administration: https://www.fda.gov/drugs/drug-safety-and-availability/questions-and-answers-risk-next-morning-impairment-after-use-insomnia-drugs-fda-requires-lower.

106 **"Of the FDA-approved drugs":** Maya Dusenbery, *Doing Harm: The Truth About How Bad Medicine and Lazy Science Leave Women Dismissed, Misdiagnosed, and Sick* (New York: HarperOne, 2018), 35. I recommend this account to anyone looking for a deeper reported dive into how medicine treats women today.

106 **failed to treat women who are sick:** Diane E. Hoffmann and Anita J. Tarzian, "The Girl Who Cried Pain: A Bias Against Women in the Treatment of Pain," *The Journal of Law, Medicine and Ethics* 29, no. 1 (2001): 13–27.

106 **women in various ERs:** Esther H. Chen et al., "Gender disparity in analgesic treatment of emergency department patients with acute abdominal pain," *Academic Emergency Medicine* 15, no. 5 (2008): 414–18.

106 **underwent cardiac catheterization:** Jacob Steenblik et al., "Gender Disparities in Cardiac Catheterization Rates Among Emergency Department Patients with Chest Pain," *Critical Pathways in Cardiology*, no. 2 (June 2021) 67—70.

107 **women wait an average of fifteen minutes longer:** From Josefina Robertson's master's thesis in medicine, "Waiting Time at the Emergency Department from a Gender Equity Perspective." See https://gupea.ub.gu.se/bitstream/2077/39196/1/gupea_2077_39196_1.pdf.

107 **treatment of women of color:** K. H. Todd et al., "Ethnicity and analgesic practice," *Annals of Emergency Medicine* 35, no. 1 (2000): 11–6, and Brandon W. Ng et al., "The influence of Latinx American identity on pain perception and treatment seeking," *Journal of Pain Research* 12 (November 2019): 3025–35; and Kevin A. Schulman et al., "The effect of race and sex on physicians' recommendations for cardiac catheterization," *The New England Journal of Medicine* 340, no. 8 (1999): 618–6.

107 **2.5 times more likely to die:** The report measured maternal outcomes in the year 2018. The full details are at https://www.cdc.gov/nchs/maternal-mortality/index.htm.

107 **It is a distinctive kind of injustice:** Miranda Fricker, "Testimonial Injustice," chapter 1 in *Epistemic Power: Power and the Ethics of Knowing* (Oxford: Oxford University Press, 2008).

108 **Ethical loneliness:** Jill Stauffer, *Ethical Loneliness: The Injustice of Not Being Heard* (New York: Columbia University Press, 2015).

109 **The notion that sick women are inventing:** Ehrenreich and English, "The Sexual Politics of Sickness," chapter 4 in *For Her Own Good*; Anne Harrington, "The Body That Speaks," chapter 2 in *The Cure Within: A History of Mind-Body Medicine* (New York: W. W. Norton, 2009).

109 **"hystera," in Greek:** H. E. Sigerist, *A History of Medicine: Primitive and Archaic Medicine* (New York: Oxford University Press, 1951).

109 **"if a physician cannot identify":** Tracey Loughran, "Hysteria and neurasthenia in pre-1914 British medical discourse and in histories of shell-shock," *History of Psychiatry* 19, no. 1 (2008): 25–46.

110 **"product and prisoner of her reproductive system":** Carroll Smith-Rosenberg and Charles Rosenberg, "The Female Animal: Medical and Biological Views of Woman and Her Role in Nineteenth-Century America," *The Journal of American History* 60, no. 2 (September 1973), 335.

110 **Psychoanalysis was the creative process:** I would be remiss if I did not note that Freud also helped decouple hysteria from gender. He wrote a paper titled "On Male Hysteria," and explored the origins of male psychic trauma such as shell shock.

111 **a patient was no longer "the best judge":** Harrington, *The Cure Within*, 76.

111 **expressing psychological distress:** See Ehrenreich and English, *For Her Own Good*; Harrington, *The Cure Within*; Dusenbery, *Doing Harm*.

112 **sites of emotional and social trauma:** See, for a brief history, Elaine Showalter, "Hysteria, Feminism, and Gender," chapter 4 in *Hysteria Beyond Freud* (Berkeley: University of California Press, 1993).

CHAPTER NINE: THE IMMUNE SYSTEM GONE AWRY

116 **go seriously awry:** Stefan H. E. Kaufmann, "Immunology's Coming of Age," *Frontiers in Immunology*, no. 10, April 2019, https://pure.mpg.de/rest/items/item_3053161/component/file_3053162/content.

119 **can affect and co-opt the immune system:** S. K. Singh and H. J. Girschick, "Lyme borreliosis: From infection to autoimmunity," *Clinical Microbiology and Infection* 10, no. 7 (2004): 598–614.

120 **sergeant cells:** Ling Lu, Joseph Barbi, and Fan Pan, "The regulation of immune tolerance by FOXP3," *Nature Reviews Immunology* 17, no. 11 (2017): 703–17. See Moises Velasquez-Manoff, *An Epidemic of Absence: A New Way of Understanding Allergies and Autoimmune Diseases* (New York: Scribner, 2012), 14.

120 **type 1 diabetes in first-generation Pakistani children:** R. G. Feltbower et al., "Trends in the incidence of childhood diabetes in south Asians and other children in Bradford, UK," *Diabetic Medicine* 19, no. 2 (2002): 162–66.

120 **"womb-to-tomb" studies:** Data show a rise not only in autoimmune disorders but allergic and atopic disease, all of which are driven by immune dysfunction. H. Okada et al., "The 'hygiene hypothesis' for autoimmune and allergic diseases: An update," *Clinical and Experimental Immunology* 160, no. 1 (2010): 1–9; Xiaofa Qin, "What caused the increase of autoimmune and allergic diseases: A decreased or an increased exposure to luminal microbial components?," *World Journal of Gastroenterology* 13, no. 8 (2007): 1306–7; J. M. Hopkin, "Mechanisms of enhanced prevalence of asthma and atopy in developed countries," *Current Opinion in Immunology* 9, no. 6 (1997): 788–92; L. C. Von Hertzen et al., "Asthma and atopy—the price of affluence?," *Allergy* 59, no. 2 (2004): 124–37; Jean-François Bach, "The effect of

infections on susceptibility to autoimmune and allergic diseases," *The New England Journal of Medicine* 347, no. 12 (2002): 911–20.

121 **"hygiene hypothesis":** D. P. Strachan, "Hay fever, hygiene, and household size," *British Medical Journal* 299, no. 6710 (1989): 1259–60.

121 **immune cells go after harmless things:** Velasquez-Manoff, *An Epidemic of Absence*, 7–8. Velasquez-Manoff builds out the evidence for the case that a decline in infectious disease is a key culprit in rising rates of autoimmune disease. He describes the work of the French scientist Jean-François Bach, who in 2002 argued that "the main factor in the increased prevalence of these diseases in industrialized countries is the reduction in the incidence of infectious diseases in those countries over the past three decades." A striking two-part graph put together by Bach shows the decline (because of vaccines) since 1950 of infectious diseases such as measles, mumps, TB, and hepatitis A in industrialized nations and what appears to be a corresponding rise in autoimmune and allergic disease. Back in 1950, thousands of people got measles and mumps; in 1980, almost no one did, but suddenly thousands of people got multiple sclerosis. Why would infection help keep inflammatory diseases in check? In the past, dangerous viruses and bacterial infections may have killed everyone in a community *except* those with mutations that made their immune system particularly active and able to fight off a disease. We are here, perhaps, because our grandparents survived cholera as a result of mutations that led them to have particularly aggressive adaptive immune responses to the dangerous infection; in this view, our forebears' genes were likely to be somewhat pro-inflammatory. In the late nineteenth and early twentieth centuries, owing to the sanitary revolution and the advent of antibiotics and vaccines, the human experience of viruses and parasites and bacteria radically changed. In a short period of time, Westerners began contracting—and living with—fewer infectious diseases. Our immune system has had almost no time to evolve in response to this radical shift, so people in Western societies are more likely to have autoimmune and allergic reactions. Or so the theory goes.

122 **the so-called leaky gut:** The rise of processed and fast food may play a specific role, too, in adding large amounts of salt to our diet. Research from Yale University in 2013 suggests that diets heavy in salt—such as the amounts found in fast food—produce an overly amped-up immune response (in the form of excessive numbers of the TH17 cell, an immune helper cell that produces inflammatory cytokines); excessive salt consumption may be a trigger for multiple sclerosis. Markus Kleinewietfeld et al., "Sodium chloride drives autoimmune disease by the induction of pathogenic TH17 cells," *Nature* 496, no. 7446 (2013).

122 **extinction of whole species of microbiota:** Justin Sonnenburg and Erica Sonnenburg, *The Good Gut: Taking Control of Your Weight, Your Mood, and Your Long-Term Health* (New York: Penguin Books, 2015).

122 **babies born by cesarean section:** Astrid Sevelsted et al., "Cesarean section and chronic immune disorders," *Pediatrics* 135, no. 1 (2015): e92–98.

122 **in the fetal-cord blood of ten newborns:** From "Body Burden: The Pollution in Newborns," a benchmark investigation of industrial chemicals, pollutants, and pesticides in umbilical cord blood from the Environmental Working Group, https://www.ewg.org/research/body-burden-pollution-newborns.

122 **study identified 55 chemicals:** Aolin Wang et al., "Suspect Screening, Prioritization, and Confirmation of Environmental Chemicals in Maternal-Newborn Pairs from San Francisco," *Environmental Science and Technology* 55, no. 8 (2021): 5037–49.

123 **an "autogenic" effect on our bodies:** Donna Jackson Nakazawa, *The Autoimmune*

Epidemic: Bodies Gone Haywire in a World Out of Balance—and the Cutting-Edge Science That Promises Hope (New York: Touchstone, 2008), chapter 2, loc. 201, Kindle.

123 **T cells of genetically susceptible mice:** Kathleen M. Gilbert, Neil R. Pumford, and Sarah J. Blossom, "Environmental Contaminant Trichloroethylene Promotes Autoimmune Disease and Inhibits T-cell Apoptosis in MRL(+/+) Mice," *Journal of Immunotoxicology* 3, no. 4 (2006): 263–67.

123 **law means that the EPA is now required:** The Frank R. Lautenberg Chemical Safety for the 21st Century Act, Pub. L. No. 114-182, 130 Stat (2016).

123 **continues to use chemicals and pesticides banned:** "US cosmetics are full of chemicals banned by Europe—why?," *The Guardian*, May 22, 2019, https://www .theguardian.com/us-news/2019/may/22/chemicals-in-cosmetics-us-restricted-eu.

124 **how the Epstein-Barr virus triggers lupus:** John B. Harley et al., "Transcription factors operate across disease loci, with EBNA2 implicated in autoimmunity," *Nature Genetics* 50, no. 5 (2018): 699–707.

126 **replicated X chromosome:** Wesley H. Brooks and Yves Renaudineau, "Epigenetics and autoimmune diseases: The X chromosome-nucleolus nexus," *Frontiers in Genetics* 6, no. 22 (February 16, 2015).

126 **estrogen interacts with the adaptive:** Christine M. Grimaldi et al., "Estrogen alters thresholds for B cell apoptosis and activation," *The Journal of Clinical Investigation* 109, no. 12 (2002): 1625–33. Some evidence suggests that estrogen allows B cells that normally would be selected for deletion to survive, possibly leading to autoimmune activity.

126 **"many autoimmune disorders tend to affect women":** Fariha Angum et al., "The Prevalence of Autoimmune Disorders in Women: A Narrative Review," *Cureus* 12, no. 5 (May 13, 2020): e8094.

127 **studies show that women are at higher risk:** Maunil K. Desai and Roberta Diaz Brinton, "Autoimmune Disease in Women: Endocrine Transition and Risk Across the Lifespan," *Frontiers in Endocrinology* 10, no. 265 (April 29, 2019).

127 **one such mechanism is "methylation":** Bilian Jin et al., "DNA methylation: Superior or subordinate in the epigenetic hierarchy?," *Genes and Cancer* 2, no. 6 (2011): 607–17.

127 **Alterations in our methylation processes:** Zimu Zhang and Rongxin Zhang, "Epigenetics in autoimmune diseases: Pathogenesis and prospects for therapy," *Autoimmunity Reviews* 14, no. 10 (2015): 854–63.

128 **While researchers take pains to distinguish:** Shanta R. Dube et al., "Cumulative childhood stress and autoimmune diseases in adults," *Psychosomatic Medicine* 71, no. 2 (2009): 243–50.

128 **how trauma and stress:** John B. Williamson et al., "Maladaptive autonomic regulation in PTSD accelerates physiological aging," *Frontiers in Psychology* 5 (January 21, 2015): 1571.

129 **"I now accept that uncertainty occupies":** Michael D. Lockshin, *The Prince at the Ruined Tower: Time, Uncertainty, and Chronic Illness* (New York: Custom Databanks, Inc., 2017), loc. 10, Kindle.

129 **"Negative Capability":** John Keats, *Selected Letters* (New York: Penguin Classics, 2015).

130 **"the vale of Soul-making":** Keats, *Selected Letters*.

CHAPTER TEN: AUTOIMMUNITY AS METAPHOR

136 **a fever scene often symbolized:** Miriam Bailin, *The Sickroom in Victorian Fiction: The Art of Being Ill* (Cambridge: Cambridge University Press, 1994), 5–47.

137 "the signal pathology": Warwick Anderson and Ian R. Mackay, *Intolerant Bodies: A Short History of Autoimmunity* (Baltimore: Johns Hopkins University Press, 2014), 8.

137 "All autoimmune diseases invoke": Sarah Manguso, *The Two Kinds of Decay* (New York: Farrar, Straus and Giroux, 2008), 1.

138 "Recognition of 'self'": F. M. Burnet, "The basis of allergic diseases," *Medical Journal of Australia* 1, no. 2 (1948): 30.

138 But along the way: Warwick Anderson, "Tolerance," *Somatosphere*, October 27, 2014, http://somatosphere.net/2014/tolerance.html/#_ftn3.

139 "is equipped with the biological equivalent": Excerpt from George Carlin's *You Are All Diseased*, HBO live broadcast stand-up special, recorded on February 6, 1999.

139 our immunity as a powerful personalized defense system: Barbara Ehrenreich, *Natural Causes: An Epidemic of Wellness, the Certainty of Dying, and Killing Ourselves to Live Longer* (New York: Twelve, 2018), loc. 45, Kindle.

140 "aiding" cancer cells "to spread": Ehrenreich, *Natural Causes*, loc. 60, Kindle.

140 Macrophages—the kind of innate immune cell: Gary Stix, "A Malignant Flame," *Scientific American*, July 1, 2008.

140 cancer as an other: In 1971, Richard Nixon signed the National Cancer Act, ushering in an era of research that became known colloquially as "a war on cancer." Perhaps that language evolved because we think of cancer as being caused by things that come from outside us—carcinogens, smoking, processed meats, the sun. Interestingly, the rise of the war on cancer in the United States followed a rise in concern about chemicals in the environment—Nixon's National Cancer Act was passed nine years after Rachel Carson's *Silent Spring* became a best seller. Then, too, cancer has a treatment, one that is usually so taxing on the body that the language of war may have evolved as a way to fortify the patient. For more, see Vincent T. DeVita, "The 'War on Cancer' and its impact," *Nature Clinical Practice Oncology* 1, no, 55 (2004).

141 "Confess your faults one to another": James 5:16 (AV). The Bible: Authorized King James Version (Oxford: Oxford World's Classics, 2008).

142 the "danger model": Polly Matzinger, "The danger model: A renewed sense of self," *Science* 296, no. 5566 (2002): 301–5.

143 "There are no incurable diseases": Bernie S. Siegel, *Love, Medicine and Miracles* (New York: HarperCollins, 1986), 99.

144 "What a grotesque being I am": Alice James, *The Diary of Alice James*, ed. Leon Edel (New York: Dodd, Mead & Company, 1964), 48.

144 "Self-disgust": W. N. P. Barbellion, *The Journal of a Disappointed Man* (1919), Project Gutenberg, final entry, https://www.gutenberg.org/files/39585/39585-h/39585-h.htm.

144 "I could feel an uneasiness deep in my bones": Norman Cousins, *Anatomy of an Illness, as Perceived by the Patient: Reflections on Healing and Regeneration* (New York: W. W. Norton, 2005).

145 "This long disease, my life": Alexander Pope, "Epistle to Dr Arbuthnot," *Alexander Pope*, ed. Pat Rogers (Oxford: Oxford University Press, 1993), 336–50, line 1734.

CHAPTER ELEVEN: MIND/BODY

147 could do real damage to the body: For an insightful review of thinking about chronic stress and the HPA axis, see "Understanding the stress response," Harvard Health Publishing, July 6, 2020, https://www.health.harvard.edu/staying-healthy/understanding-the-stress-response.

148 **cortisol levels spike:** Ji-Won Chun et al., "Role of Frontostriatal Connectivity in Adolescents with Excessive Smartphone Use," *Frontiers in Psychiatry* 9, no. 437 (September 12, 2018).

149 **Sleep deprivation can impair functioning:** A. M. Williamson and A. M. Feyer, "Moderate sleep deprivation produces impairments in cognitive and motor performance equivalent to legally prescribed levels of alcohol intoxication," *Occupational and Environmental Medicine* 57, no. 10 (2000): 649–55.

149 **chronically sleep deprived:** Janet M. Mullington et al., "Cardiovascular, inflammatory, and metabolic consequences of sleep deprivation," *Progress in Cardiovascular Diseases* 51, no. 4 (2009): 294–302.

149 **parts of our brains connected to fear:** M. Spreng, "Possible health effects of noise induced cortisol increase," *Noise and Health* 2, no. 7 (2000): 59–64.

149 **The World Health Organization recommends a maximum threshold:** "WHO recommends setting night noise limits at 40 decibels," European Commission DG ENV News Alert, issue 202, July 1, 2020, https://ec.europa.eu/environment /integration/research/newsalert/pdf/202na3_en.pdf.

149 **"the thousand intricate problems":** S. Weir Mitchell, *Wear and Tear: Or, Hints for the Overworked* (New York: Arno Press, 1973. First published by J. B. Lippincott Company, 1871).

149 **diagnosing an epidemic of hysteria:** Julie Beck, "Americanitis," *The Atlantic*, March 11, 2016, https://www.theatlantic.com/health/archive/2016/03/the-history -of-neurasthenia-or-americanitis-health-happiness-and-culture/473253/.

149 **emotions could affect the body's physiology:** I rely partly on Robert M. Sapolsky's *Why Zebras Don't Get Ulcers: The Acclaimed Guide to Stress, Stress-Related Diseases, and Coping* (New York: Macmillan, 2004) for my history of modern thinking about stress.

151 **process that led to the animals' disease:** Many years later, Selye said if he had understood English better, he would have said these demands cause "strain," since all living "stresses" the body, not all of it negatively.

151 **hardening of the arteries:** Andrew Steptoe and Mika Kivimäki, "Stress and cardiovascular disease," *Nature Reviews Cardiology* 9, no. 6 (2012): 360–70.

151 **illnesses like irritable bowel syndrome worse:** E. J. Bennett et al., "Level of chronic life stress predicts clinical outcome in irritable bowel syndrome," *Gut* 43, no. 2 (1998): 256–61, https://www.ncbi.nlm.nih.gov/pmc/articles/PMC1727204/pdf/v04 3p00256.pdf.

151 **can lead to dysfunction in cortisol production:** Kara E Hannibal and Mark D. Bishop, "Chronic stress, cortisol dysfunction, and pain: A psychoneuroendocrine rationale for stress management in pain rehabilitation," *Physical Therapy* 94, no. 12 (2014): 1816–25.

151 **immune system becomes *more active*:** Selye was correct to say that ultimately for most people stress lowers immunity—it inhibits production of immune cells, makes it hard to produce antibodies, and impairs the communication that calls immune cells to the site of injury or infection. How does this happen? The adrenal gland releases chemicals called "glucocorticoids," which are the body's own steroid hormones— including cortisol. They suppress production of immune cells by shrinking the thymus gland where T cells are produced and inhibiting the release of other chemicals that communicate with circulating lymphocytes, so that your white blood cells are less likely to hear an "alarm" that an infection is present. Experiments have shown that the immune system can be suppressed "independently of glucocorticoid secretion strongly implicating these other routes," Sapolsky notes; it appears that the sympathetic nervous system and the pituitary play a role in the suppression of immunity,

too. Long-term major stresses leave the immune system significantly suppressed, but episodic stress appears to follow an up-and-down pattern.

152 **"repeated ups and downs":** Sapolsky, *Why Zebras Don't Get Ulcers*, 159. (See chapter 8, "Immunity, Stress, and Disease," for an extended discussion.)

153 **and poorer maternal outcomes:** A. T. Geronimus, "The weathering hypothesis and the health of African-American women and infants: Evidence and speculations," *Ethnicity and Disease* 2, no. 3 (Summer 1992): 207–21, PMID 1467758.

153 **structural insecurity lead to telomere shortening:** Telomeres are repeated sequences of DNA at the ends of chromosomes that function like sticky caps or the plastic at the ends of shoelaces; DNA strands get shorter with each cell replication, but telomeres help prevent key information from being lost. Research suggests that telomere shortening is a key factor in how we age; the process of shortening can speed up or slow down depending on lifestyle choices. (Smoking and UV light exposure, for example, are thought to hasten telomere shortening.)

153 **social, interconnected nature of our bodies:** See Arline T. Geronimus et al., "'Weathering' and age patterns of allostatic load scores among blacks and whites in the United States," *American Journal of Public Health* 96, no. 5 (2006): 826–33.

CHAPTER TWELVE: POSITIVE THINKING

155 **"What seemed inexcusable":** Norman Cousins, *Anatomy of an Illness, as Perceived by the Patient: Reflections on Healing and Regeneration* (New York: W. W. Norton, 2005), 31.

156 **determinants of cancer:** See Anne Harrington, *The Cure Within: A History of Mind-Body Medicine* (New York: W. W. Norton, 2009), 198–204, and Robert M. Sapolsky, *Why Zebras Don't Get Ulcers: The Acclaimed Guide to Stress, Stress-Related Diseases, and Coping* (New York: Macmillan, 2004), 175–78.

157 **live longer than the women in the control group:** David Spiegel et al., "Effect of psychosocial treatment on survival of patients with metastatic breast cancer," *The Lancet* 334, no. 8668 (1989): 888–91.

157 **The "pinkwashing" of breast cancer:** Anne Boyer, *The Undying* (New York: Farrar, Straus and Giroux, 2019).

157 **failed to replicate his results:** See David Spiegel et al., "Effects of supportive-expressive group therapy on survival of patients with metastatic breast cancer: A randomized prospective trial," *Cancer* 110, no. 5 (2007): 1130–38. In *Why Zebras Don't Get Ulcers*, Robert Sapolsky observes that a possible explanation for Spiegel's findings was that the group therapy support, in an era when a cancer diagnosis was often kept a secret, made cancer patients more likely to complete their chemotherapy regimens and take their medications. Evidence shows that about 25 percent of patients, he reports, miss chemo sessions or skip other medications, because the treatment is so challenging. The support from group therapy may have encouraged more compliance, and thus better outcomes. (Today, he points out, nearly all patients get the benefit of social support, because hospitals have in-house therapy programs and a cancer diagnosis is typically no longer a secret, making the study hard to replicate.) Sapolsky, *Why Zebras Don't Get Ulcers*, 176–78.

158 **positive thinking does not lead to better outcomes:** James C. Coyne and Howard Tennen, "Positive psychology in cancer care: Bad science, exaggerated claims, and unproven medicine," *Annals of Behavioral Medicine* 39, no. 1 (2010): 16–26.

158 **little to do with each other:** Benjamin E. Steinberg et al., "Bacteria and the Neural Code," *The New England Journal of Medicine* 371 (2014): 2131–33.

158 **experiment about behavioral conditioning:** My discussion of Ader's experiment is drawn from Harrington, *The Cure Within*, chapter 3, "The Power of Positive Thinking," 126–27, and Sapolsky, *Why Zebras Don't Get Ulcers*, chapter 8, "Immunity, Stress, and Disease," 143–44.

159 **"a psychological 'prime'":** Bruce Grierson, "What if Age Is Nothing but a Mind-Set?," *The New York Times Magazine*, October 22, 2014.

159 **the men's sight and hearing had improved:** Ellen Langer, *Counterclockwise: Mindful Health and the Power of Possibility* (New York: Ballantine Books, 2009).

160 **but the simulator was broken:** Ellen Langer et al., "Believing Is Seeing: Using Mindlessness (Mindfully) to Improve Visual Acuity," *Psychological Science* 21, no. 5 (May 2010): 661–66.

160 **startling impact for the management of type 2 diabetes:** Chanmo Park et al., "Blood glucose level in diabetes and perceived time," *Proceedings of the National Academy of Sciences* 113, 29 (July 2016): 8168–70.

162 **more vulnerable than they did without one:** Nortin Hadler, *Worried Sick: A Prescription for Health in an Overtreated America* (Chapel Hill: University of North Carolina Press, 2008), 39.

162 **"The flip side of positivity":** Barbara Ehrenreich, *Bright-Sided: How Positive Thinking Is Undermining America* (New York: Metropolitan Books, 2009), 8.

162 **One mother of a son with cancer:** Harrington, *The Cure Within*, 198.

162 **"Cancer cells are internalized anger":** Barbara Boggs Sigmund, "I Didn't Give Myself Cancer," *The New York Times*, December 30, 1989.

CHAPTER THIRTEEN: POSSIBILITY

165 **I published an article about my experience:** Meghan O'Rourke, "What's Wrong with Me?," *The New Yorker*, August 26, 2013, https://www.newyorker.com/magazine/2013/08/26/whats-wrong-with-me.

168 **vitamin D has an immunomodulatory effect:** Low levels of serum vitamin D are prevalent in several autoimmune diseases, including lupus and MS among others. Environmental and genetic factors may be implicated (some evidence suggests that sick people go outside less, but evidence also suggests that genetic polymorphisms, or mutation, lead to low vitamin D levels associated with autoimmune disease). See Chen-Yen Yang et al., "The implication of vitamin D and autoimmunity: A comprehensive review," *Clinical Reviews in Allergy and Immunology* 45, no. 2 (2013): 217–26.

168 **a boost of endorphins can help modulate:** For evidence about LDN's effects, see Jarred Younger et al., "The use of low-dose naltrexone (LDN) as a novel anti-inflammatory treatment for chronic pain," *Clinical Rheumatology* 33, no. 4 (2014): 451–59. Also J. Wybran, "Enkephalins and endorphins as modifiers of the immune system: Present and future," *Federation Proceedings* 44, no. 1, pt. 1 (1985): 92–94.

172 **didn't want to prescribe antibiotics:** See this 2020 report on the CDC's standard test: https://www.lymedisease.org/study-cdcs-two-tier-lyme-testing-was-inaccurate-in-more-than-70-of-cases/.

172 **try a phosphatidylcholine drip:** "Phosphatidylcholine," RxList, reviewed June 11, 2021. For more about phosphatidylcholine and its uses, see https://www.rxlist.com/phosphatidylcholine/supplements.htm.

174 **pricked by the poisoned gom jabbar:** Frank Herbert, *Dune* (New York: Ace Books, 2003), 10–15.

CHAPTER FOURTEEN: NADIR

179 **"decided to get rid of the notebook":** William Styron, *Darkness Visible* (New York: Vintage, 1992), 59.

184 **doesn't reimburse patients for ozone therapy:** For more on ozone and ultraviolet irradiation treatments, see Michael R. Hamblin, "Ultraviolet Irradiation of Blood: 'The Cure That Time Forgot?,'" *Advances in Experimental Medicine and Biology* 996 (2017): 295–309.

186 **an "art monster":** Jenny Offill, *Dept. of Speculation* (New York: Vintage, 2014).

187 **"I, in my soul, am alive too":** John Ashbery, "A Blessing in Disguise," in *Rivers and Mountains* (New York: Holt, Rinehart, and Winston, 1966).

190 **overseeing Lyme grants:** See Mary Beth Pfeiffer, "The Battle over Lyme Disease: Is It Chronic?," *Poughkeepsie Journal*, March 26, 2014.

CHAPTER FIFTEEN: LYME DISEASE

191 **arranged in mandalas:** This chapter relies on my article "Lyme Disease Is Baffling, Even to Experts," from *The Atlantic*, September 2019. For that article, I conducted extensive reporting and interviews with the CDC, Allen Steere, Brian Fallon, Monica Embers, Paul Auwaerter, Kim Lewis, Richard Horowitz, Richard Ostfeld, and many more, and the material here was checked with the participants.

192 **doctors should use their judgment:** See "Lyme Disease: Diagnosis and Testing," Centers for Disease Control and Prevention, https://www.cdc.gov/lyme/diagnosis testing/index.html; and Paul Mead, Jeannine Petersen, and Alison Hinkley, "Updated CDC Recommendation for Serologic Diagnosis of Lyme Disease," *Morbidity and Mortality Weekly Report* 68 (2019): 703, https://www.cdc.gov/mmwr/volumes /68/wr/mm6832a4.htm?s_cid=mm6832a4_w, for evolving CDC recommendations around Lyme disease testing. See also A. Moore, C. A. Nelson, C. Molins, et al., "Current Guidelines, Common Clinical Pitfalls, and Future Directions for Laboratory Diagnosis of Lyme Disease, United States," *Emerging Infectious Diseases* 22, no. 7 (2016): 1169–77, https://wwwnc.cdc.gov/eid/article/22/7/15-1694_article, for information about the two-tiered serologic test and the 1994 agreement; for the CDC-approved recommendations that grew out of the 1994 conference, see Centers for Disease Control and Prevention, "Recommendations for test performance and interpretation from the Second National Conference on Serologic Diagnosis of Lyme Disease," *Morbidity and Mortality Weekly Report* 44, no. 31 (1995): 590–91.

193 **the Lyme bacterium:** The role of co-infections in PTLDS and chronic Lyme disease is understudied, even as studies suggest that *Babesia microti*, for example, is a growing risk: see Michelle H. Hersh et al., "Co-infection of blacklegged ticks with *Babesia microti* and *Borrelia burgdorferi* is higher than expected and acquired from small mammal hosts," *PloS ONE* 9, no. 6 (June 18, 2014); and Gary P. Wormser et al., "Co-infections in Persons with Early Lyme Disease, New York, USA," *Emerging Infectious Diseases* 25, no. 4 (2019): 748–52.

194 **cases increased almost fivefold:** See "Lyme Disease: Data and Surveillance," Centers for Disease Control and Prevention, https://www.cdc.gov/lyme/datasurveil lance/index.html, and "Lyme Disease Data Tables: Historical Data," Centers for Disease Control and Prevention, https://www.cdc.gov/lyme/stats/tables.html.

194 **a significant concern for the national blood supply:** "Babesiosis and the U.S. blood supply," https://www.cdc.gov/parasites/babesiosis/resources/babesiosis_policy_brief .pdf.

195 **now prevalent in Northern California:** See "Lyme Disease Maps: Most Recent Year," Centers for Disease Control and Prevention, https://www.cdc.gov/lyme /datasurveillance/maps-recent.html, and "Lyme Borreliosis in Europe," European Centre for Disease Prevention and Control, https://www.ecdc.europa.eu/sites /portal/files/media/en/healthtopics/vectors/world-health-day-2014/Documents /factsheet-lyme-borreliosis.pdf.

196 **still cannot be prevented by a vaccine:** For more information, see "Valneva and Pfizer Announce Initiation of Phase 2 Study for Lyme Disease Vaccine Candidate," Valneva, March 8, 2021, https://valneva.com/press-release/valneva-and-pfizer -announce-initiation-of-phase-2-study-for-lyme-disease-vaccine-candidate/.

196 **black-legged ticks that live on mice:** Interviews and emails with Allen Steere, March–July 2019.

196 **researchers describe it as an "immune evader":** See medical literature on *Borrelia*'s "immune evasion" and "immune escape" strategies, such as Bilal Aslam et al., "Immune escape strategies of *Borrelia burgdorferi*," *Future Microbiology* 2 (October 2017): 1219–37.

197 **can make its way into fluid in the joints:** See Norbert Scheffold et al., "Lyme carditis—Diagnosis, Treatment and Prognosis," *Deutsches Arzteblatt International* 112, no. 12 (2015): 202–8. The CDC website discusses Lyme carditis as well: https://www.cdc.gov/lyme/treatment/lymecarditis.html. Also the CDC on neurological cases of Lyme disease: https://www.cdc.gov/lyme/treatment/Neurologic Lyme.html.

197 **doxycycline for patients with early Lyme:** The 2019 updated IDSA guidelines can be found here: https://www.idsociety.org/practice-guideline/lyme-disease/. The 2006 IDSA guidelines: Gary P. Wormser et al., "The clinical assessment, treatment, and prevention of Lyme disease, human granulocytic anaplasmosis, and babesiosis: Clinical practice guidelines by the Infectious Diseases Society of America," *Clinical Infectious Diseases* 43, no. 9 (2006): 1089–134.

197 **medical system's seeming inability to help:** This history is drawn from personal interviews in 2016 and 2019 with Brian Fallon; Elizabeth Maloney, the president of the Partnership for Tick-Borne Diseases Education and ILADS board member; Paul Auwaerter; Allen Steere; as well as my reading of contemporaneous Lyme disease news articles from 1979 on.

198 **Lyme infections could leave people sick for years:** Interview with Elizabeth Maloney, July 2019; also see the 2014 ILADS guidelines, found here: Daniel J. Cameron, Lorraine B. Johnson, and Elizabeth L. Maloney, "Evidence assessments and guideline recommendations in Lyme disease: The clinical management of known tick bites, erythema migrans rashes and persistent disease," *Expert Review of Anti-Infective Therapy* 12, no. 9 (2014): 1103–35.

198 **was a pseudoscientific diagnosis:** Personal interview and emails with Allen Steere, March–July 2019; Steere referred to the notion that many people with systemic PTLDS/chronic Lyme disease who improve on antibiotics may have another medical condition but are captive to what he called a "Lyme disease ideology." It is possible that antibiotics help them because of the placebo effect, or perhaps because of a similar bacterial infection for which, as he put it, Lyme disease can serve "as a model" (in the sense that it existed for years before medical science knew what it was).

198 **patient in her thirties died:** Natalie S. Marzec et al., "Serious Bacterial Infections Acquired During Treatment of Patients Given a Diagnosis of Chronic Lyme Disease—United States," *Morbidity and Mortality Weekly Report* 66, no. 23 (2017): 607–9.

199 **experts in the IDSA camp implied:** See, for instance, David Grann, "Stalking Dr. Steere," *The New York Times Magazine,* June 17, 2001.

199 **IDSA guidelines for patients and physicians included the warning:** Wormser et al., "The clinical assessment, treatment, and prevention of Lyme disease, human granulocytic anaplasmosis, and babesiosis," 1115. As the 2006 IDSA guidelines put it, "In many patients, posttreatment symptoms appear to be more related to the aches and pains of daily living rather than to either Lyme disease or a tickborne coinfection. Put simply, there is a relatively high frequency of the same kinds of symptoms in 'healthy' people. For example, 20 percent to 30 percent of adults complain of chronic fatigue, and in the 2003 National Health Interview Survey, the frequency of doctor-diagnosed arthritis cases among adults was 21.5 percent. A study in England found a point prevalence of 11.2 percent for the presence of self-reported chronic widespread pain among adults that was frequently associated with feelings of depression and anxiety, fatigue, and somatic symptoms. A recent study of the general adult United States population estimated a point prevalence of self-reported serious pain (level 3) to be 3.75 percent to 12.10 percent, depending on the assessment tool used; for level 3 emotional or cognitive dysfunction, it was 2.17 percent to 3.42 percent. Population-based surveillance in the United States indicates a mean of 6.1 self-reported unhealthy days during the preceding month. Thus, the presence of arthralgia, myalgia, fatigue, and other subjective symptoms after treatment for Lyme disease must be evaluated in the context of 'background' complaints in a significant proportion of individuals."

200 **"postural orthostatic tachycardia syndrome":** Some studies connect POTS both to autoimmune disease and to infectious triggers; for example, see William T. Gunning III et al., "Postural Orthostatic Tachycardia Syndrome Is Associated with Elevated G-Protein Coupled Receptor Autoantibodies," *Journal of the American Heart Association* (September 2019).

201 **patients can experience some blend of fatigue:** My description of POTS is taken from many sources, but mainly interviews with Amy Kontorovich, a genetic cardiologist at Mount Sinai, and Ruwanthi Titano, a cardiologist specializing in post-COVID care of POTS, in November and December 2020. There is a helpful introduction to it on the Johns Hopkins Medicine page: https://www.hopkinsmedi cine.org/health/conditions-and-diseases/postural-orthostatic-tachycardia -syndrome-pots. Johns Hopkins also has one of the few treatment centers dedicated to POTS: https://www.hopkinsmedicine.org/physical_medicine_rehabilitation /services/programs/pots/.

204 **Sue Visser, the CDC's associate director for policy:** For more on chronic Lyme and PTLDS, see Adriana Marques, "Chronic Lyme Disease: A Review," *Infectious Disease Clinics of North America* 22, no. 2 (2008): 341–60, https://www.sciencedirect .com/science/article/abs/pii/S0891552007001274?via%3Dihub. See also Alison W. Rebman et al., "The Clinical, Symptom, and Quality-of-Life Characterization of a Well-Defined Group of Patients with Posttreatment Lyme Disease Syndrome," *Frontiers in Medicine* 4, no. 224 (December 2017).

204 **little federal funding to study Lyme disease:** As of 2019, the NIH spent only $768 on each new confirmed case of Lyme, compared to $36,063 on each new case of hepatitis C; see Tick-Borne Disease Working Group, *2018 Report to Congress* (Washington, DC: U.S. Department of Health and Human Services, 2018), 3, https://www.hhs.gov/sites/default/files/tbdwg-report-to-congress-2018.pdf. Things are finally beginning to change: in fiscal year 2021, the federal government has committed to $91 million in funding for Lyme disease research, up

from just $55 million the year before; see https://www.lymedisease.org/historic
-increase-in-lyme-funding/. Even so, much of the money to investigate PTLDS
has come from private foundations, as noted in the text. In 2019, the CDC and
the NIH reached out to these groups, officials told me, spurred in part by the
2018 Tick-Borne Disease Working Group report to Congress outlining major gaps
in the scientific understanding of Lyme disease; interview with the CDC, July 2019.

205 **in patients who developed PTLDS:** John Aucott, personal interview. See also
Lisa K. Blum et al., "Robust B Cell Responses Predict Rapid Resolution of Lyme
Disease," *Frontiers in Immunology* 9, no. 1634 (July 2018), and Marije Oosting et al.,
"Functional and Genomic Architecture of *Borrelia burgdorferi*–Induced Cytokine
Responses in Humans," *Cell Host and Microbe* 20, no. 6 (2016): 822–33.

206 **macaques had varying immune responses to the infection:** Monica E. Embers
et al., "Persistence of *Borrelia burgdorferi* in rhesus macaques following antibiotic
treatment of disseminated infection," *PloS ONE* 7, no. 1 (2012): e29914.

206 *Borrelia* **spirochetes in the brain and central nervous system:** Shiva Kumar Goud
Gadila et al., "Detecting *Borrelia* Spirochetes: A Case Study with Validation Among
Autopsy Specimens," *Frontiers in Neurology* 12, no. 628045 (May 2021): 707, and
https://news.tulane.edu/pr/study-finds-evidence-persistent-lyme-infection
-brain-despite-aggressive-antibiotic-therapy.

207 **"We now have not only a plausible explanation":** Jie Feng et al., "Stationary phase
persister/biofilm microcolony of *Borrelia burgdorferi* causes more severe disease in a
mouse model of Lyme arthritis: Implications for understanding persistence, Post-
treatment Lyme Disease Syndrome (PTLDS), and treatment failure," *Discovery
Medicine* 27, no. 148 (2019): 125–38.

209 **"A virus is the most likely candidate":** Boyce Rensberger, "A New Type of Arthritis
Found in Lyme," *The New York Times*, July 18, 1976, https://www.nytimes.com
/1976/07/18/archives/a-new-type-of-arthritis-found-in-lyme-new-form-of-arthritis
-is.html.

210 **"Nothing is more threatening":** Atul Gawande, *Being Mortal: Medicine and What
Matters in the End* (New York: Metropolitan Books, 2014), 4.

CHAPTER SIXTEEN: FUTURITY

211 **felt nothing like an American medical office:** See the Taymount Clinic website at
https://taymount.com/.

212 **suggests a genetic tendency:** Huihui Xu et al., "The Dynamic Interplay Between
the Gut Microbiota and Autoimmune Diseases," *Journal of Immunology Research*
2019, no. 7546047 (October 27, 2019), and F. De Luca and Y. Shoenfeld, "The
microbiome in autoimmune diseases," *Clinical and Experimental Immunology* 195,
no. 1 (2019): 74–85.

215 **"Our gut is home":** Justin Sonnenburg and Erica Sonnenburg, *The Good Gut: Taking Control of Your Weight, Your Mood, and Your Long-Term Health* (New York: Penguin Books, 2015).

215 **increased rates of asthma and weakened immune response:** Simone Becattini, Ying
Taur, and Eric G. Palmer, "Antibiotic-Induced Changes in the Intestinal Microbi-
ota and Disease," *Trends in Molecular Medicine* 22, no. 6 (2016): 458–78; Cecilia
Jernberg et al., "Long-term ecological impacts of antibiotic administration on the
human intestinal microbiota," *ISME Journal* 1, no. 1 (2007): 56–66; and Hadar
Neuman et al., "Antibiotics in early life: Dysbiosis and the damage done," *FEMS
Microbiology Reviews* 42, no. 4 (2018): 489–99.

215 **Fewer strains of microbes:** Melanie Schirmer et al., "Linking the Human Gut Microbiome to Inflammatory Cytokine Production Capacity," *Cell* 167, no. 4 (2016): 1125–36, e8.

216 **FMT was so effective:** Els van Nood et al., "Duodenal infusion of donor feces for recurrent *Clostridium difficile,*" *The New England Journal of Medicine* 368, no. 5 (2013): 407–15.

216 **screen and freeze donor material to send to doctors and hospitals:** "OpenBiome," Center for Microbiome Informatics and Therapeutics, https://microbiome.mit.edu /our-ecosystem/openbiome/. In 2019, one man with a *C. diff* infection died after receiving an FMT supplied by OpenBiome before undergoing a bone-marrow transplant, which underscored that the procedure is not without risks.

216 **Studies in humans have had dramatic results:** L. Desbonnet et al., "Effects of the probiotic *Bifidobacterium infantis* in the maternal separation model of depression," *Neuroscience* 170, no. 4 (2010): 1179–88.

217 **subjects who took the GOS:** Kristin Schmidt et al., "Prebiotic intake reduces the waking cortisol response and alters emotional bias in healthy volunteers," *Psychopharmacology* 232, no. 10 (2015): 1793–801.

217 **connection between bacteria we eat and our brain function:** Kirsten Tillisch et al., "Consumption of fermented milk product with probiotic modulates brain activity," *Gastroenterology* 144, no. 7 (2013): 1394–401, 1401.e1–4.

220 **which FMT helps with:** As Enid Taylor of the Taymount Clinic was careful to point out, an FMT can also produce short-term inflammation; a person with inflammatory bowel disease should do an FMT only when the disease is in remission or being managed with medication.

222 **threat to some pregnancies:** M. D. Lockshin, "Pregnancy Loss and Antiphospholipid Antibodies," *Lupus* 7, no. 2 suppl. (February 1998): 86–89.

222 **My doctor put me on steroids:** For more on the possible benefits of IVIG treatment in patients with autoimmune disease and pregnancy loss, see Tal Sapir et al., "Intravenous Immunoglobulin (IVIG) as Treatment for Recurrent Pregnancy Loss (RPL)," *Harefuah* 144, no. 6 (2005): 415–20, 453, 454; and D. D. Kiprov et al., "The use of intravenous immunoglobulin in recurrent pregnancy loss associated with combined alloimmune and autoimmune abnormalities," *American Journal of Reproductive Immunology* 36, no. 4 (1996): 228–34.

CHAPTER EIGHTEEN: SILENCE AND HEALING

236 **needed less pain medication:** R. S. Ulrich, "View through a window may influence recovery from surgery," *Science* 224, no. 4647 (1984): 420–21. See also Esther M. Sternberg, *Healing Spaces: The Science of Place and Well-Being* (Cambridge, MA: Belknap Press, 2009), loc. 19, Kindle. I rely on Sternberg's book for much of my discussion of healing spaces in this chapter.

237 **His work on lupus vulgaris:** From *Nobel Lectures, Physiology or Medicine 1901–1921* (Amsterdam: Elsevier Publishing Company, 1967); see Niels Ryberg Finsen– Biographical, Nobel Prize Outreach AB 2021, August 14, 2021, https://www .nobelprize.org/prizes/medicine/1903/finsen/biographical; italics in Finsen quote are in the original.

237 **"By the late twentieth century, state-of-the-art hospitals":** Sternberg, *Healing Spaces*, loc. 39, Kindle.

238 **"In palliative care":** Sternberg, *Healing Spaces*, loc. 3195, Kindle.

238 **effect of a Quaker meeting:** George Prochnik, *In Pursuit of Silence: Listening for Meaning in a World of Noise* (New York: Doubleday, 2010), loc. 68, Kindle.

238 **Donne was fifty-one:** My account of John Donne and his illness is drawn from John Stubbs's *John Donne: The Reformed Soul* (New York: W. W. Norton, 2008), 399–405.

239 **"a part of the main":** John Donne, *Devotions upon Emergent Occasions* (New York: Vintage, 1999).

CHAPTER NINETEEN: SOLUTIONS

242 **"The world can't afford regular sympathy":** Hermione Lee introduction to Virginia Woolf, *On Being Ill* (Ashfield, MA: Paris Press, 2002), xxviii.

242 **"Those great wars which the body wages":** Woolf, *On Being Ill*, 5.

247 **The quest at Mount Sinai's Center:** "Center for Post-COVID Care," Mount Sinai, https://www.mountsinai.org/about/covid19/center-post-covid-care. Some of the material about long COVID is based on my original reporting for *The Atlantic* on the establishment of post-COVID centers, in which I followed doctors and patients in real time as they struggled to understand and then treat long COVID: "Unlocking the Mysteries of Long COVID," *The Atlantic*, April 2021.

248 **was a puzzling group:** The data in this paragraph come from interviews with Zijian Chen, David Putrino, Dayna McCarthy, Ruwanthi Titano, and more, November 2020–January 2021.

249 **usually triggered by mental or physical exertion:** Hannah E. Davis et al., "Characterizing Long COVID in an International Cohort: 7 Months of Symptoms and Their Impact," medRxiv (2020), https://www.medrxiv.org/content/10.1101/2020 .12.24.20248802v2; *EClinicalMedicine*, 101019 (July 2021). Note that some respondents in this group had never received positive COVID tests, given how hard tests were to come by in the early months of the pandemic in the spring of 2020.

249 **10 to 30 percent of those infected with the novel coronavirus:** This figure is based on interviews with the teams at Mount Sinai. See also Jennifer K. Logue et al., "Sequelae in Adults at 6 Months After COVID-19 Infection," *JAMA Network Open* 4, no. 2 (2021): e210830. And this early report on long COVID: Angelo Carfì et al., "Persistent Symptoms in Patients After Acute COVID-19," *The Journal of the American Medical Association* 324, no. 6 (2020): 603–5.

250 **getting vaccinated resolved their symptoms:** See Tim Gruber, "Some Long Covid Patients Feel Much Better After Getting Vaccine," *The New York Times*, March 17, 2021, https://www.nytimes.com/2021/03/17/health/coronavirus-patients-and -vaccine-effects.html; and Melba Newsome, "Could the COVID-19 Vaccine Help Long-Hauler Symptoms?," AARP, May 26, 2021, https://www.aarp.org/health /conditions-treatments/info-2021/vaccines-may-help-long-haulers-covid.html.

251 **publicly recognized long COVID:** "NIH launches new initiative to study 'Long COVID,'" National Institutes of Health, February 23, 2021, https://www.nih.gov /about-nih/who-we-are/nih-director/statements/nih-launches-new-initiative -study-long-covid.

254 **These centers could be:** For example, some patients whose symptoms don't resolve after an infection turn out also to have Ehlers-Danlos syndrome (a set of genetic connective tissue disorders); some have food sensitivities; others have mold exposure; still others may have craniocervical instability (CCI), a condition that can result in pathological compression of the brain stem or spinal cord. Receiving a diagnosis of and treatment for CCI has helped some people with ME go into remission. See, for example, Jennifer Brea's posts on Medium about her CCI diagnosis and treatment: https://jenbrea.medium.com/cci-tethered-cord-series-e1e098b5edf.

CHAPTER TWENTY: THE WISDOM NARRATIVE

258 "Life is not just a question of courage": Susan Sontag, *Alice in Bed* (New York: Farrar, Straus and Giroux, 1993), 68.

258 able to handle their illness with "grace": Arthur Kleinman, *The Illness Narratives: Suffering, Healing, and the Human Condition* (New York: Basic Books, 1989).

258 "Unmaking can be a generative process": Arthur Frank, *The Wounded Storyteller* (Chicago: University of Chicago Press, 2013), loc. 2733, Kindle. I rely in this chapter on this astute and insightful book, mainly for its understanding of the kinds of stories that sick people tell themselves.

260 "*repair* the damage": Frank, *The Wounded Storyteller*, chapter 1, loc. 214–23, Kindle.

260 "Contemporary culture treats health": Frank, *The Wounded Storyteller*, loc. 1325, Kindle.

260 health care workers interpreted his experiences: Frank, *The Wounded Storyteller*, loc. 83, Kindle.

260 "events are told as the storyteller experiences life": Frank, *The Wounded Storyteller*, loc. 1620, Kindle.

260 borrows from the legal philosopher Ronald Dworkin: Frank, *The Wounded Storyteller*, loc. 980, Kindle. Ronald Dworkin, *Life's Dominion: An Argument About Abortion, Euthanasia, and Individual Freedom* (New York: Alfred A. Knopf, 1993), 211.

261 "searching for alternative ways of being ill": Frank, *The Wounded Storyteller*, loc. 1918, Kindle.

261 who suffered from debilitating headaches: Friedrich Nietzsche, *The Gay Science: With a Prelude in Rhymes and an Appendix of Songs*, trans. with commentary by Walter Kaufmann (New York: Vintage, 1974), 249–90.

261 "battle of being mortal": Atul Gawande, *Being Mortal: Medicine and What Matters in the End* (New York: Metropolitan Books, 2014), 139–40.

261 "It's bearable, and yet *I cannot bear it*": Alphonse Daudet, *In the Land of Pain*, trans. Julian Barnes (New York: Alfred A. Knopf, 2003), 9.

262 The quest "is always an education": Alasdair MacIntyre, *After Virtue: A Study in Moral Theory* (Notre Dame, IN: University of Notre Dame Press, 1981), 219.

263 "wisdom-talk is big business in America": Jennifer Ratner-Rosenhagen, "A Mind of One's Own," *Dissent*, Fall 2015.

264 "One of our most difficult duties": Frank, *The Wounded Storyteller*, loc. 579, Kindle.

264 the self in relation to others: Frank, *The Wounded Storyteller*, loc. 710, Kindle.

265 I found myself thinking of James Joyce's story: James Joyce, "The Dead," in *Dubliners*, ed. Jeri Johnson (Oxford: Oxford University Press, 2008), 176.

266 "My visions of a future": Audre Lorde, *The Cancer Journals* (San Francisco: Aunt Lute Books, 1980), 15.

267 "I would lie if I did not also speak of loss": Lorde, *The Cancer Journals*, 16.

267 "camouflaged grieving": Jennifer Stitt, "Will COVID-19 Strengthen Our Bonds?," *Guernica*, May 12, 2020.

267 "standing for what one was meant to stand for": Alice James, *The Death and Letters of Alice James: Selected Correspondence*, ed. Ruth Yeazell (Berkeley: The University of California Press, 1981), 34.

BIBLIOGRAPHY

Author's note: I consulted more texts than are represented here, but since such a list would be unwieldy, I've included a list of those I quote or found instrumental to the development of my thinking on the subjects I discuss in this book.

Alsan, Marcella, and Marianne Wanamaker. "Tuskegee and the Health of Black Men." *The Quarterly Journal of Economics* 133, no. 1 (February 2018), 407–55.

American Autoimmune Related Diseases Association and National Coalition of Autoimmune Patient Groups. *The Cost Burden of Autoimmune Disease: The Latest Front in the War on Healthcare Spending*. Eastpointe, MI: American Autoimmune Related Diseases Association, 2011.

Anderson, Gerard. *Chronic Conditions: Making the Case for Ongoing Care*. Princeton, NJ: Robert Wood Johnson Foundation, 2004, https://www.giaging.org/documents/509 68chronic.care.chartbook.pdf.

Anderson, Warwick. "Tolerance." *Somatosphere* (October 27, 2014), http://somatosphere .net/2014/tolerance.html/#_ftn3.

Anderson, Warwick, and Ian R. Mackay. *Intolerant Bodies: A Short History of Autoimmunity*. Baltimore: Johns Hopkins University Press, 2014.

Angum, Fariha, Tahir Khan, Jasndeep Kaler, et al. "The Prevalence of Autoimmune Disorders in Women: A Narrative Review." *Cureus* 12, no. 5 (May 2020), e8094.

Aronowitz, Robert A. "Lyme Disease: The Social Construction of a New Disease and Its Social Consequences." *The Milbank Quarterly* 69, no. 1 (1991), 79–112.

Ashbery, John. *The Double Dream of Spring*. New York: Ecco, 1976.

———. *Rivers and Mountains*. New York: Ecco, 1966.

Aslam, Bilal, Muhammad Atif Nisar, Mohsin Khurshid, and Muhammad Khalid Farooq Salamat. "Immune Escape Strategies of *Borrelia burgdorferi*." *Future Microbiology* 12 (October 2017), 1219–37.

Bach, Jean-François. "The Effect of Infections on Susceptibility to Autoimmune and Allergic Diseases." *The New England Journal of Medicine* 347, no. 12 (September 2002), 911–20.

Bailey, Patricia Hill. "The Dyspnea-Anxiety-Dyspnea Cycle—COPD Patients' Stories of Breathlessness: 'It's Scary / When You Can't Breathe.'" *Qualitative Health Research* 14, no. 6 (July 2004), 760–78.

Bailin, Miriam. *The Sickroom in Victorian Fiction: The Art of Being Ill.* Cambridge: Cambridge University Press, 1994.

Bair, Barbara, and Susan E. Cayleff, eds. *Wings of Gauze: Women of Color and the Experience of Health and Illness.* Detroit: Wayne State University Press, 1993.

Barbellion, W. N. P. *The Journal of a Disappointed Man.* With an introduction by H. G. Wells. New York: George H. Doran, 1919.

Barnes, David S. *The Making of a Social Disease: Tuberculosis in Nineteenth-Century France.* Berkeley: University of California Press, 1995.

Bauman, Zygmunt. *Mortality, Immortality, and Other Life Strategies.* Stanford, CA: Stanford University Press, 1992.

Beard, Charles B., Rebecca J. Eisen, Christopher M. Barker, et al. "Vector Borne Diseases." In *The Impacts of Climate Change on Human Health in the United States: A Scientific Assessment.* Washington, DC: U.S. Global Change Research Program, 2016, 129–56.

Beauchamp, Tom L. "Informed Consent: Its History, Meaning, and Present Challenges." *Cambridge Quarterly of Healthcare Ethics* 20, no. 4 (August 2011), 515–23.

Becattini, Simone, Ying Taur, and Eric G. Pamer. "Antibiotic-Induced Changes in the Intestinal Microbiota and Disease." *Trends in Molecular Medicine* 22, no. 6 (June 2016), 458–78.

Beck, Julie. "'Americanitis': The Disease of Living Too Fast." *The Atlantic* (March 11, 2016), https://www.theatlantic.com/health/archive/2016/03/the-history-of-neurasthenia-or-americanitis-health-happiness-and-culture/473253/.

Beckman, Howard B., and Richard M. Frankel. "Academia and Clinic: The Effect of Physician Behavior on the Collection of Data." *Annals of Internal Medicine* 101 (1984), 692–96.

Bennett, E. J., C. C. Tennant, C. Piesse, et al. "Level of Chronic Life Stress Predicts Clinical Outcome in Irritable Bowel Syndrome." *Gut* 43 (1998), 256–61.

Benvenga, Salvatore, and Fabrizio Guarneri. "Molecular mimicry and autoimmune thyroid disease." *Reviews in Endocrine and Metabolic Disorders* 17, no. 4 (2016), 485–98.

Bhatt, Jay, and Priya Bathija. "Ensuring Access to Quality Health Care in Vulnerable Communities." *Academic Medicine* 93, no. 9 (2018), 1271–75.

Biss, Eula. *On Immunity: An Inoculation.* Minneapolis: Graywolf Press, 2014.

Blum, Lisa K., Julia Z. Adamska, Dale S. Martin, et al. "Robust B Cell Responses Predict Rapid Resolution of Lyme Disease." *Frontiers in Immunology* 18, no. 9 (July 2018), 1634.

Boyer, Anne. *The Undying.* New York: Farrar, Straus and Giroux, 2019.

Brea, Jennifer, director. *Unrest.* Shella Films, 2017.

Brooks, Wesley H., and Yves Renaudineau. "Epigenetics and Autoimmune Diseases: The X Chromosome–Nucleolus Nexus." *Frontiers in Genetics* 6 (February 2015), 22.

Broyard, Anatole. *Intoxicated by My Illness.* New York: Fawcett, 1993.

Bugiardini, Raffaele, Jinsung Yoon, Sasko Kedev, et al. "Prior Beta-Blocker Therapy for Hypertension and Sex-Based Differences in Heart Failure Among Patients with Incident Coronary Heart Disease." *Hypertension: Journal of the American Heart* 76 (2020), 819–26.

Burnet, F. M. "The basis of allergic diseases." *Medical Journal of Australia* 1, no. 2 (1948), 29–35.

Cameron, Daniel J., Lorraine B. Johnson, and Elizabeth L. Maloney. "Evidence Assessments and Guideline Recommendations in Lyme Disease: The Clinical Management of Known Tick Bites, Erythema Migrans Rashes and Persistent Disease." *Expert Review of Anti-Infective Therapy* 12, no. 9 (September 2014), 1103–35.

Campbell, Colin, and Gill McGauley. "Doctor-Patient Relationships in Chronic Illness: Insights from Forensic Psychiatry." *British Medical Journal* 330, no. 7492 (March 2005), 667–70.

Carfi, Angelo, Roberto Bernabei, and Francesco Landi. "Persistent Symptoms in Patients After Acute COVID-19." Research Letter. *The Journal of the American Medical Association* 324, no. 6 (2020), 603–5.

Carlin, George. *You Are All Diseased.* HBO live broadcast stand-up special. New York, Beacon Theater. Recorded February 6, 1999.

Carstensen, Laura. "Aging, Emotion, and Health-Related Decision Strategies: Motivational Manipulations Can Reduce Age Differences." *Psychology and Aging* 22, no. 1 (2007), 134–46.

———. "Growing Old or Living Long: Take Your Pick." *Issues in Science and Technology* 23, no. 2 (January 2007), 41–50.

———. "Older People Are Happier." TEDxWomen 2011 (December 2011), https://www.ted.com/talks/laura_carstensen_older_people_are_happier.

Centers for Disease Control and Prevention. "Babesiosis and the U.S. Blood Supply." Center for Global Health, Division of Parasitic Diseases and Malaria (July 15, 2013), https://www.cdc.gov/parasites/babesiosis/resources/babesiosis_policy_brief.pdf.

———. "Lyme Disease Maps: Most Recent Year." Lyme Disease, Recent Surveillance Data (2019), https://www.cdc.gov/lyme/datasurveillance/maps-recent.html.

———. "Recommendations for Test Performance and Interpretation from the Second National Conference on Serologic Diagnosis of Lyme Disease." *Morbidity and Mortality Weekly Report* 44, no. 31 (1995), 590–91.

Chang, Kiki, Harold S. Koplewicz, and Ron Steingard. "Special Issue on Pediatric Acute-Onset Neuropsychiatric Syndrome." *Journal of Child and Adolescent Psychopharmacology* 25, no. 1 (February 2015), 1–2.

Charmaz, Kathy. "Loss of Self: A Fundamental Form of Suffering in the Chronically Ill." *Sociology of Health and Illness* 5, no. 2 (1983), 168–95.

Chen, Daniel C. R., Daniel S. Kirshenbaum, Jun Yan, et al. "Characterizing Changes in Student Empathy Throughout Medical School." *Medical Teaching* 34, no. 4 (2012), 305–11.

Chen, Esther H., Frances S. Shofer, Anthony J. Dean, et al. "Gender Disparity in Analgesic Treatment of Emergency Department Patients with Acute Abdominal Pain." *Academic Emergency Medicine* 15, no. 5 (May 2008), 414–18.

Chun, Ji-Won, Jihye Choi, Hyun Cho, et al. "Role of Frontostriatal Connectivity in Adolescents with Excessive Smartphone Use." *Frontiers in Psychiatry* 9 (2018), 437.

Cochran, Jack, and Charles C. Kenney. *The Doctor Crisis: How Physicians Can, and Must, Lead the Way to Better Health Care.* New York: PublicAffairs, 2014.

Committee on the Diagnostic Criteria for Myalgic Encephalomyelitis/Chronic Fatigue Syndrome, Institute of Medicine of the National Academies. *Beyond Myalgic Encephalomyelitis/Chronic Fatigue Syndrome: Redefining an Illness.* Washington, DC: The National Academies Press, forthcoming.

Committee on Understanding the Biology of Sex and Gender Differences, Institute of Medicine. *Exploring the Biological Contributions to Human Health: Does Sex Matter?* Washington, DC: National Academies Press, 2001.

Cousins, Norman. *Anatomy of an Illness, as Perceived by the Patient: Reflections on Healing and Regeneration.* New York: W. W. Norton, 2005.

Coyne, James C., and Howard Tennen. "Positive Psychology in Cancer Care: Bad Science, Exaggerated Claims, and Unproven Medicine." *Annals of Behavioral Medicine* 39, no. 1 (2010), 16–26.

Crosby, Christina. *A Body, Undone.* New York: New York University Press, 2016.

Cutler, David. *The Quality Cure: How Focusing on Health Care Quality Can Save Your Life and Lower Spending Too.* Berkeley: University of California Press, 2014.

Daudet, Alphonse. *In the Land of Pain.* Translated by Julian Barnes. New York: Alfred A. Knopf, 2003.

Davis, Hannah E., Gina S. Assaf, Lisa McCorkell, et al. "Characterizing Long COVID in an International Cohort: 7 Months of Symptoms and Their Impact." EClinicalMedicine, published by *The Lancet* 101019 (July 15, 2021).

Deen, Gibrilla F., Nathalie Broutet, Wenbo Xu, et al. "Ebola RNA Persistence in Semen of Ebola Virus Disease Survivors—Final Report." *The New England Journal of Medicine* 377 (October 12, 2017), 1428–37.

Del Canale, Stefano, Daniel Z. Louis, Vittorio Maio, et al. "The Relationship Between Physician Empathy and Disease Complications: An Empirical Study of Primary Care Physicians and Their Diabetic Patients in Parma, Italy." *Academic Medicine* 87, no. 9 (September 2012), 1243–49.

De Luca, F., and Y. Shoenfeld. "The Microbiome in Autoimmune Diseases." *Clinical and Experimental Immunology* 195, no. 1 (January 2019), 74–85.

Derksen, Frans, Jozien Bensing, and Antoine Lagro-Janssen. "Effectiveness of Empathy in General Practice: A Systematic Review." *British Journal of General Practice* 63, no. 606 (January 2013), 76–84.

Desai, Maunil K., and Roberta Diaz Brinton. "Autoimmune Disease in Women: Endocrine Transition and Risk Across the Lifespan." *Frontiers in Endocrinology* 10 (2019), 1–19.

DeSalle, Rob, and Susan L. Perkins. *Welcome to the Microbiome: Getting to Know the Trillions of Bacteria and Other Microbes In, On, and Around You.* With illustrations by Patricia J. Wynne. New Haven, CT: Yale University Press, 2015.

DeVita, Vincent T., Jr. "The 'War on Cancer' and Its Impact." *Nature Clinical Practice Oncology* 1 (2004), 55.

Dhakal, Aayush, and Evelyn Sbar. "Jarisch Herxheimer Reaction." *StatPearls* (May 4, 2021), https://ncbi.nlm.nih.gov/books/NBK557820/.

Diagnostic and Statistical Manual of Mental Disorders (DSM-III). 3rd edition. Washington, DC: American Psychiatric Association, 1980.

Dinse, Gregg E., Christine G. Parks, Clarice R. Weinberg, et al. "Increasing Prevalence of Antinuclear Antibodies in the United States." *Arthritis and Rheumatology* 72, no. 6 (June 2020), 1026–35.

Donne, John. *Devotions upon Emergent Occasions and Death's Duel.* With *The Life of Dr. John Donne* by Izaak Walton. Preface by Andrew Motion. New York: Vintage, 1999.

Douthat, Ross. *The Deep Places: A Memoir of Illness and Discovery.* New York: Convergent, 2021.

Dube, Shanta R., DeLisa Fairweather, William S. Pearson, et al. "Cumulative Childhood Stress and Autoimmune Diseases in Adults." *Psychosomatic Medicine* 71, no. 2 (February 2009), 243–50.

Dusenbery, Maya. *Doing Harm: The Truth About How Bad Medicine and Lazy Science Leave Women Dismissed, Misdiagnosed, and Sick.* New York: HarperOne, 2018.

Dworkin, Ronald. *Life's Dominion: An Argument About Abortion, Euthanasia, and Individual Freedom.* New York: Alfred A. Knopf, 1993.

Ehrenreich, Barbara. *Bright-Sided: How Positive Thinking Is Undermining America.* New York: Metropolitan Books, 2009.

———. *Natural Causes: An Epidemic of Wellness, the Certainty of Dying, and Killing Ourselves to Live Longer.* New York: Twelve, 2018.

Ehrenreich, Barbara, and Deirdre English. *For Her Own Good: Two Centuries of the Experts' Advice to Women.* New York: Anchor Books, 2005.

Eiser, Arnold R. *The Ethos of Medicine in Postmodern America.* Washington, DC: Lexington Books, 2013.

Embers, Monica E., Stephen W. Barthold, Juan T. Borda, et al. "Persistence of *Borrelia burgdorferi* in Rhesus Macaques Following Antibiotic Treatment of Disseminated Infection." *PLoS ONE* 7, no. 1 (2012), 1–12.

Environmental Working Group. "Body Burden: The Pollution in Newborns" (July 14, 2005), https://www.ewg.org/research/body-burden-pollution-newborns.

European Commission Directorate-General for Environment News Alert Service. "WHO Recommends Setting Night Noise Limits at 40 Decibels." *Science for Environment Policy* 202 (July 1, 2020), https://ec.europa.eu/environment/integration /research/newsalert/pdf/202na3_en.pdf.

Fasano, Alessio. "Leaky gut and autoimmune diseases." *Clinical Reviews in Allergy and Immunology* 42, no. 1 (2012).

Feltbower, R. G., H. J. Bodansky, P. A. McKinney, et al. "Trends in the Incidence of Childhood Diabetes in South Asians and Other Children in Bradford, UK." *Diabetic Medicine* 19, no. 2 (February 2002), 162–66.

Feng, Jie, Tingting Li, Rebecca Yee, et al. "Stationary Phase Persister/Biofilm Microcolony of *Borrelia burgdorferi* Causes More Severe Disease in a Mouse Model of Lyme Arthritis: Implications for Understanding Persistence, Post-Treatment Lyme Disease Syndrome (PTLDS), and Treatment Failure." *Discovery Medicine* 27, no. 148 (March 2019), 125–38.

Frank, Arthur W. *The Wounded Storyteller: Body, Illness, and Ethics.* 2nd edition. Chicago: University of Chicago Press, 2013.

Fricker, Miranda. *Epistemic Injustice: Power and the Ethics of Knowing.* Oxford: Oxford University Press, 2007.

Gadila, Shiva Kumar Goud, Gorazd Rosoklija, Andrew J. Dwork, et al. "Detecting *Borrelia* Spirochetes: A Case Study with Validation Among Autopsy Specimens." *Frontiers in Neurology* 12 (May 2021), 1–14.

García-Gómez, Elizabeth, Edgar Ricardo Vázquez-Martínez, Christian Reyes-Mayoral, et al. "Regulation of Inflammation Pathways and Inflammasome by Sex Steroid Hormones in Endometriosis." *Frontiers in Endocrinology* 10, no. 935 (January 2020), 1–17.

Garfield, Sidney R. "The Delivery of Medical Care." *Scientific American* 222 (April 1970), 15–23.

Gawande, Atul. *Being Mortal: Medicine and What Matters in the End.* New York: Metropolitan Books, 2014.

Gelder, M. G. "Neurosis: Another Tough Old Word." *British Medical Journal* (Clinical Research Edition) 292, no. 6526 (April 1986), 972–73.

Geronimus, A. T. "'Weathering' and Age Patterns of Allostatic Load Scores Among Blacks and Whites in the United States." *American Journal of Public Health* 95, no. 5 (2006), 826–33.

———. "The Weathering Hypothesis and the Health of African-American Women and Infants: Evidence and Speculations." *Ethnicity and Disease* 2, no. 3 (Summer 1992), 207–21.

Gilbert, Kathleen M., Neil R. Pumford, and Sarah J. Blossom. "Environmental Contaminant Trichloroethylene Promotes Autoimmune Disease and Inhibits T-cell Apoptosis in MRL(+/+) Mice." *Journal of Immunotoxicology* 3, no. 4 (December 2006), 263–67.

Gilman, Charlotte Perkins. "The Yellow Wall-Paper." In *The Yellow Wall-Paper, Herland, and Selected Writings.* New York: Penguin Books, 1999, 166–82.

Gilman, Sander L., Helen King, Roy Porter, et al. *Hysteria Beyond Freud.* Berkeley and Los Angeles: University of California Press, 1993.

Grann, David. "Stalking Dr. Steere." *The New York Times Magazine* (June 17, 2001), https://www.nytimes.com/2001/06/17/magazine/stalking-dr-steere.html.

Green, Harvey. *Fit for America: Health, Fitness, Sport, and American Society.* New York: Pantheon, 1986.

Grierson, Bruce. "What if Age Is Nothing but a Mind-Set?" *The New York Times Magazine* (October 22, 2014), https://www.nytimes.com/2014/10/26/magazine/what-if-age-is-nothing-but-a-mind-set.html.

Gunderman, Richard. "Illness as Failure: Blaming Patients." *The Hastings Center Report* 30, no. 4 (July-August 2000), 7–11.

Hadler, Nortin M. *Worried Sick: A Prescription for Health in an Overtreated America.* Chapel Hill: University of North Carolina Press, 2008.

Hadler, Nortin M., and Susan Greenhalgh. "Labeling Woefulness: The Social Construction of Fibromyalgia." *Spine* 30, no. 1 (2004), 1–4.

Hall, William J., Mimi V. Chapman, Kent M. Lee, et al. "Implicit Racial/Ethnic Bias Among Health Care Professionals and Its Influence on Health Care Outcomes: A Systematic Review." *American Journal of Public Health* 105, no. 12 (December 2015), 60–76.

Hamberg, Katarina. "Gender Bias in Medicine." *Women's Health* 4, no. 3 (May 2008), 237–43.

Hamblin, Michael R. "Ultraviolet Irradiation of Blood: 'The Cure That Time Forgot'?" *Advances in Experimental Medicine and Biology* 996 (September 2017), 295–309.

Hannibal, Kara E., and Mark D. Bishop. "Chronic Stress, Cortisol Dysfunction, and Pain: A Psychoneuroendocrine Rationale for Stress Management in Pain Rehabilitation." *Physical Therapy* 94, no. 12 (December 2014), 1816–25.

Harley, John B., Xiaoting Chen, Mario Pujato, et al. "Transcription factors operate across disease loci, with EBNA2 implicated in autoimmunity." *Nature Genetics* 50, no. 5 (May 2018), 699–707.

Harvard Health Publishing, "Understanding the Stress Response" (July 6, 2020), https://www.health.harvard.edu/staying-healthy/understanding-the-stress-response.

Hemingway, Ernest. *The Sun Also Rises.* New York: Scribner, 2014.

Herbert, Frank. *Dune.* New York: Ace Books, 2003.

Herbert, George. "The Flower." In *The Poetical Works of George Herbert.* New York: George Bell and Sons, 1886.

Hersh, Michelle H., et al. "Co-infection of blacklegged ticks with *Babesia microti* and *Borrelia burgdorferi* is higher than expected and acquired from small mammal hosts." *PloS ONE* 9, no. 6 (June 18, 2014).

Hoffmann, Diane E., and Anita J. Tarzian. "The Girl Who Cried Pain: A Bias Against Women in the Treatment of Pain." *The Journal of Law, Medicine and Ethics* 29, no. 1 (Spring 2001), 13–27.

Hojat, Mohammadreza, Michael J. Bergare, Kaye Maxwell, et al. "The Devil Is in the Third Year: A Longitudinal Study of Empathy in Medical School." *Academy of Medicine* 84, no. 9 (September 2009), 1182–91.

Hojat, Mohammadreza, Salvatore Mangione, Thomas J. Nasca, et al. "An Empirical Study of Decline in Empathy in Medical School." *Medical Education* 38, no. 9 (September 2004), 934–41.

Holt, Terrence. *Internal Medicine: A Doctor's Stories.* New York: Liveright, 2015.

Hopkins, J. M. "Mechanisms of Enhanced Prevalence of Asthma and Atopy in Developed Countries." *Current Opinion in Immunology* 9, no. 6 (December 1997), 788–92.

Horowitz, Richard I. *How Can I Get Better? An Action Plan for Treating Resistant Lyme and Chronic Disease.* New York: St. Martin's Griffin, 2017.

James, Alice. *The Death and Letters of Alice James.* Edited by Ruth Bernard Yeazell. Berkeley and Los Angeles: University of California Press, 1983.

———. *The Diary of Alice James.* Edited by Leon Edel. New York: Dodd, Mead & Company, 1964.

Jauhar, Sandeep. *Doctored: The Disillusionment of an American Physician.* New York: Farrar, Straus and Giroux, 2014.

Jernberg, Cecilia, Soja Löfmark, Charlotta Edlund, and Janet K. Jansson. "Long-Term Ecological Impacts of Antibiotic Administration on the Human Intestinal Microbiota." *The ISME Journal* 1, no. 1 (May 2007), 56–66.

Jin, Bilian, Yajun Li, and Keith D. Robertson. "DNA Methylation: Superior or Subordinate in the Epigenetic Hierarchy?" *Genes and Cancer* 2, no. 6 (June 2011), 607–17.

Johnson, Nathanael. "Forget the Placebo Effect: It's the 'Care Effect' That Matters." *Wired* (January 18, 2013), https://www.wired.com/2013/01/dr-feel-good/.

———. *All Natural: A Skeptic's Quest for Health and Happiness in an Age of Ecological Anxiety.* Emmaus, PA, and New York: Rodale Books, 2013.

Joyce, James. "The Dead." In *Dubliners.* Edited by Jeri Johnson. Oxford: Oxford University Press, 2008, 138–76.

Kaakinen, Pirjo, Maria Kääriäinen, and Helvi Kyngäs. "The chronically ill patients' quality of counselling in the hospital." *Journal of Nursing Education and Practice* 2, no. 4 (November 2012), 114–23.

Kaptchuk, Ted J., John M. Kelley, Lisa A. Conboy, et al. "Components of Placebo Effect: Randomised Controlled Trial in Patients with Irritable Bowel Syndrome." *British Medical Journal* (Clinical Research Edition) 336, no. 7651 (May 2008), 999–1003.

Karr-Morse, Robin, and Meredith S. Wiley. *Scared Sick: The Role of Childhood Trauma in Adult Disease.* New York: Basic Books, 2012.

Kayser, Matthew S., and Josep Dalmau. "The emerging link between autoimmune disorders and neuropsychiatric disease." *The Journal of Neuropsychiatry and Clinical Neurosciences* 23, no. 1 (2011), 90–97.

Keats, John. *Selected Letters.* Edited by John Barnard. New York: Penguin Classics, 2015.

Khakpour, Porochista. *Sick: A Memoir.* New York: Harper Perennial, 2018.

Kiprov, D. D., R. D. Nachtigall, R. C. Weaver, et al. "The Use of Intravenous Immunoglobulin in Recurrent Pregnancy Loss Associated with Combined Alloimmune and Autoimmune Abnormalities." *American Journal of Reproductive Immunology* 36, no. 4 (October 1996), 228–34.

Kleinewietfeld, Markus, Arndt Manzel, Jens Titze, et al. "Sodium Chloride Drives Autoimmune Disease by the Induction of Pathogenic TH16 Cells." *Nature* 496, no. 7446 (April 2013), 518–22.

Kleinman, Arthur. *The Illness Narratives: Suffering, Healing and the Human Condition.* New York: Basic Books, 1989.

Knoff, William F. "A History of the Concept of Neurosis, with a Memoir of William Cullen." *American Journal of Psychiatry* 127, no. 1 (July 1970), 120–24.

Langer, Ellen J. *Counterclockwise: Mindful Health and the Power of Possibility.* New York: Ballantine Books, 2009.

Langer, Ellen, Maja Djikic, Michael Pirson, et al. "Believing Is Seeing: Using Mindlessness (Mindfully) to Improve Visual Acuity." *Psychological Science* 21, no. 5 (May 2010), 661–66.

Laurence, Leslie, and Beth Weinhouse. *Outrageous Practices: How Gender Bias Threatens Women's Health.* New Brunswick, NJ: Rutgers University Press, 1997.

Lavine, Elana. "Blood testing for sensitivity, allergy or intolerance to food." *Canadian Medical Association Journal* 184, no. 6 (2012), 666–68.

L'Engle, Madeleine. *A Wind in the Door.* New York: Dell, 1980.

Lerner, Barron H. *The Good Doctor: A Father, a Son, and the Evolution of Medical Ethics.* New York: Beacon Press, 2014.

Levy, Deborah. *The Cost of Living: An Autobiography.* New York: Bloomsbury, 2019.

Lewis, Sinclair. *Arrowsmith.* New York: New American Library, 2011.

Li, Qian-Qian, et al. "Acupuncture effect and central autonomic regulation." *Evidence-based Complementary and Alternative Medicine: eCAM* 2013 (2013), 267959.

Lockshin, Michael D. "Pregnancy Loss and Antiphospholipid Antibodies." *Lupus* 7, no. 2 (February 1998), 86–89.

———. *The Prince at the Ruined Tower: Time, Uncertainty, and Chronic Illness.* New York: Custom Databanks, Inc., 2017.

Logue, Jennifer K., Nicholas M. Franko, and Denise J. McCulloch. "Sequelae in Adults at 6 Months After COVID-19 Infection." *JAMA Network Open* 4, no. 2 (February 19, 2021).

Lorde, Audre. *The Cancer Journals.* San Francisco: Aunt Lute Books, 1980.

Lu, L., J. Barbi, and F. Pan. "The regulation of immune tolerance by FOXP3." *Nature Reviews Immunology* 17 (2017), 703–17.

MacIntyre, Alasdair. *After Virtue: A Study in Moral Theory.* 3rd edition. Notre Dame, IN: University of Notre Dame Press, 2007.

Main, T. F. "The Ailment." *British Journal of Medical Psychology* 30, no. 3 (September 1975), 129–45.

Makary, Martin A., and Michael Daniel. "Medical error—the third leading cause of death in the US," *British Medical Journal* 353 (2016), i2139.

Manguso, Sarah. *The Two Kinds of Decay.* New York: Farrar, Straus and Giroux, 2008.

Marzec, Natalie S., Christina Nelson, Paul Ravi Waldron, et al. "Serious Bacterial Infections Acquired During Treatment of Patients Given a Diagnosis of Chronic Lyme Disease—United States." *Morbidity and Mortality Weekly Report* 66, no. 23 (June 16, 2017), 607–9.

Matzinger, Polly. "The Danger Model: A Renewed Sense of Self." *Science* 296, no. 5566 (April 2002), 301–5.

McEwen, B. S. "Stress, Adaptation and Disease: Allostasis and Allostatic Load." *Annals of the New York Academy of Sciences* 840 (May 1998), 33–44.

McEwen, B. S., and Eliot Stellar. "Stress and the Individual: Mechanisms Leading to Disease." *Archives of Internal Medicine* 153, no. 18 (September 1993), 2093–101.

"Medicine and Medical Science: Black Lives Must Matter More." *The Lancet* 395 (June 13, 2020), 1813.

Mitchell, S. Weir. *Wear and Tear: Or, Hints for the Overworked.* New York: Arno Press, 1973. First published by J. B. Lippincott Company, 1871.

Monmaney, Terence. "Marshall's Hunch." *The New Yorker* (September 12, 1993), 64–72.

Moore, Andrew, Christina Nelson, Claudia Molins, et al. "Current Guidelines, Common Clinical Pitfalls, and Future Directions for Laboratory Diagnosis of Lyme Disease, United States." *Emerging Infectious Diseases* 22, no. 7 (July 2016), 1169–77.

Moseley, J. Bruce, Kimberley O'Malley, Nancy J. Petersen, et al. "A Controlled Trial of Arthroscopic Surgery for Osteoarthritis of the Knee." *The New England Journal of Medicine* 347 (July 11, 2002), 81–88.

Mullington, Janet M., Monika Haack, Maria Toth, et al. "Cardiovascular, Inflammatory, and Metabolic Consequences of Sleep Deprivation." *Progress in Cardiovascular Diseases* 51, no. 4 (January-February 2009), 294–302.

Nakazawa, Donna Jackson. *The Autoimmune Epidemic: Bodies Gone Haywire in a World Out of Balance—and the Cutting-Edge Science That Promises Hope.* New York: Touchstone, 2008.

National Institutes of Health Autoimmune Diseases Coordinating Committee. *Progress in Autoimmune Diseases Research: Report to Congress.* Washington, DC: U.S. Department of Health and Human Services and National Institutes of Health, March 2005.

Neuman, Hadar, Paul Forsythe, Atara Uzan, et al. "Antibiotics in Early Life: Dysbiosis and the Damage Done." *FEMS Microbiology Reviews* 42, no. 4 (July 2018), 489–99.

Neumann, Melanie, Friedrich Edelhäuser, Diethard Tauschel, et al. "Empathy Decline and Its Reasons: A Systematic Review of Studies with Medical Students and Residents." *Academic Medicine* 86, no. 8 (August 2011), 996–1009.

Ng, Brandon W., Namrata Nanavaty, and Vani A. Mathur. "The Influence of Latinx American Identity on Pain Perception and Treatment Seeking." *Journal of Pain Research* 12 (2019), 3025–35.

Nietzsche, Friedrich. *The Gay Science: With a Prelude in Rhymes and an Appendix of Songs.* Translated with commentary by Walter Kaufmann. New York: Vintage, 1974.

Nnoaham, Kelechi E., Lone Hummelshoj, Premila Webster, et al. "Impact of Endometriosis on Quality of Life and Work Productivity: A Multicenter Study Across Ten Countries." *Fertility and Sterility* 96, no. 2 (August 2011), 366–73.

Nobel Lectures, Physiology or Medicine 1901–1921. Amsterdam: Elsevier Publishing Company, 1967; Niels Ryberg Finsen—Biographical. NobelPrize.org, Nobel Prize Outreach AB 2021. August 14, 2021, https://www.nobelprize.org/prizes/medicine/1903/finsen/biographical.

Noble, Bill, David Clark, Marcia Meldrum, et al. "The Measurement of Pain, 1945–2000." *Journal of Pain and Symptom Management* 29, no. 1 (January 2005), 14–20.

Obenchain, Theodore G. *Genius Belabored: Childbed Fever and the Tragic Life of Ignaz Semmelweis.* Tuscaloosa: University of Alabama Press, 2016.

Offill, Jenny. *Dept. of Speculation.* New York: Vintage, 2014.

Ofri, Danielle. *What Doctors Feel: How Emotions Affect the Practice of Medicine.* Boston: Beacon Press, 2014.

———. "When the Patient Is 'Non-Compliant.'" *Well* (blog). *The New York Times* (November 15, 2012), https://well.blogs.nytimes.com/2012/11/15/when-the-patient-is-noncompliant/.

Okada, H., C. Kuhn, H. Feillet, and J.-F. Bach. "The 'Hygiene Hypothesis' for Autoimmune and Allergic Diseases: An Update." *Clinical and Experimental Immunology* 160, no. 1 (April 2010), 1–9.

Oosting, Marije, Mariska Kerstholt, Rob ter Horst, et al. "Functional and Genomic Architecture of *Borrelia burgdorferi*-Induced Cytokine Responses in Humans." *Cell Host and Microbiome* 20, no. 6 (December 2016), 822–33.

"OpenBiome." Center for Microbiome Informatics and Therapeutics, Massachusetts Institute of Technology (2012), https://microbiome.mit.edu/our-ecosystem/open biome/.

O'Rourke, Meghan. *The Long Goodbye: A Memoir*. New York: Riverhead Books, 2011.

———. "What's Wrong with Me?" *The New Yorker* (August 26, 2013), https://www .newyorker.com/magazine/2013/08/26/whats-wrong-with-me\.

Park, Chanmo, Francesco Pagnini, Andrew Reece, et al. "Blood Sugar Level Follows Perceived Time Rather Than Actual Time in People with Type 2 Diabetes." *Proceedings of the Natural Academy of Sciences in the United States of America* 113, no. 29 (July 19, 2016), 8168–70.

Park, Jinbin. "Historical Origins of the Tuskegee Experiment: The Dilemma of Public Health in the United States." *Korean Journal of Medical History: Ui Sahak* 26, no. 3 (December 2017), 545–78.

Paul, William E. *Immunity*. Baltimore: Johns Hopkins University Press, 2015.

Pavlíčková, J., J. Zbíral, M. Smatanová, et al. "Uptake of Thallium from Artificially Contaminated Soils by Kale (*Brassica oleracea* L. var. *acephala*)." *Plant, Soil and Environment* 52, no. 12 (December 2006), 544–49.

Peabody, Francis W. "The Care of the Patient." *The Journal of the American Medical Association* 88, no. 12 (1927), 877–82.

Peterson, Laurie. "Live from Davos: Aetna CEO on Health, Reinvention, and Yoga." *Yahoo News* (January 22, 2014), https://news.yahoo.com/2014-01-22-live-from-davos -aetna-ceo-on-health-reinvention-and-yoga-vide.html.

Pfeiffer, Mary Beth. "The Battle over Lyme Disease: Is It Chronic?" *Poughkeepsie Journal* (May 30, 2015), https://www.poughkeepsiejournal.com/story/news/health/lyme -disease/2014/03/26/so-called-lyme-wars/6907209/.

Philpott, Tom. "Sorry, Foodies: We're About to Ruin Kale." *Mother Jones* (July 15, 2015), https://www.motherjones.com/food/2015/07/kale-silent-killer/.

Pope, Alexander. "Epistle to Dr. Arbuthnot." In *Alexander Pope*. Edited by Pat Rogers. Oxford: Oxford University Press, 1993, 336–50.

Prochnik, George. *In Pursuit of Silence: Listening for Meaning in a World of Noise*. New York: Doubleday, 2010.

Qin, Xiaofa. "What Caused the Increase of Autoimmune and Allergic Diseases: A Decreased or an Increased Exposure to Luminal Microbial Components?" *World Journal of Gastroenterology* 13, no. 8 (February 2007), 1306–7.

Rabin, Roni Caryn. "Health Researchers Will Get $10.1 Million to Counter Gender Bias in Studies." *The New York Times* (September 23, 2014), https://www.nytimes .com/2014/09/23/health/23gender.html.

———. "Trial of Chelation Therapy Shows Benefits, but Doubts Persist." *Well* (blog). *The New York Times* (April 15, 2013), https://well.blogs.nytimes.com/2013/04/15 /trial-of-chelation-therapy-shows-benefits-but-doubts-persist/.

Ratner-Rosenhagen, Jennifer. "A Mind of One's Own." *Dissent* (Fall 2015), https:// www.dissentmagazine.org/article/mind-ones-own-feminist-wisdom.

Rebman, Alison W., Kathleen T. Bechtold, Ting Yang, et al. "The Clinical, Symptom, and Quality-of-Life Characterization of a Well-Defined Group of Patients with Posttreatment Lyme Disease Syndrome." *Frontiers in Medicine* (December 14, 2017), https://www.frontiersin.org/articles/10.3389/fmed.2017.00224/full.

Rehmeyer, Julie, *Through the Shadowlands: A Science Writer's Odyssey into an Illness Science Doesn't Understand*. Emmaus, PA: Rodale Press, 2017.

Rensberger, Boyce. "A New Type of Arthritis Found in Lyme." *The New York Times* (July 18, 1976), https://www.nytimes.com/1976/07/18/archives/a-new-type-of-arthritis -found-in-lyme-new-form-of-arthritis-is.html.

Rosen, George. "What Is Social Medicine? A Genetic Analysis of the Concept." *Bulletin of the History of Medicine* 21 (1947), 674–733.

Rosenberg, Charles E. "Back to the Future." *The Lancet* 382, no. 9895 (September 2013), 851–52.

———. *Our Present Complaint: American Medicine, Then and Now.* Baltimore: Johns Hopkins University Press, 2007.

Sacks, Oliver. *A Leg to Stand On.* New York: Summit Books, 1984.

Sapir, T., H. Carp, and Y. Shoefeld. "Intravenous Immunoglobulin (IVIG) as Treatment for Recurrent Pregnancy Loss (RPL)." *Harefuah* 144, no. 6 (2005), 415–20.

Sapolsky, Robert M. *Why Zebras Don't Get Ulcers: The Acclaimed Guide to Stress, Stress-Related Diseases, and Coping.* 3rd edition. New York: Macmillan, 2004.

Sarno, John. *Healing Back Pain: The Mind-Body Connection.* New York: Grand Central Publishing, 1991.

———. *The Mindbody Prescription: Healing the Body, Healing the Pain.* New York: Grand Central Publishing, 1998.

Scarry, Elaine. *The Body in Pain: The Making and Unmaking of the World.* Oxford: Oxford University Press, 1987.

Scheffold, Norbert, Bernhard Herkommer, Reinhard Kandolf, and Andreas E. May. "Lyme Carditis—Diagnosis, Treatment and Prognosis." *Deutsches Arzteblatt International* 112, no. 12 (March 2015), 202–8.

Schulman, Kevin A., Jesse A. Berlin, William Harless, et al. "The Effect of Race and Sex on Physicians' Recommendations for Cardiac Catheterization." *The New England Journal of Medicine* 340 (February 25, 1999), 618–26.

Schulte, Margaret F. "Editorial." *Frontiers of Health Services Management* 29, no. 4 (Summer 2013), 1–2.

Sevelsted, Astrid, Jakob Stokholm, Klaus Bønnelykke, and Hans Bisgaard. "Cesarean Section and Chronic Immune Disorders." *Pediatrics* 135, no. 1 (2015), 92–98.

Shah, Neil D., and Michael W. Fried. "Treatment Options of Patients with Chronic Hepatitis C Who Have Failed Prior Therapy." *Clinical Liver Disease* 7, no. 2 (February 2016), 40–44.

Shaw, George Bernard. *The Doctor's Dilemma.* London: Penguin New Edition, 1987.

Sheng, Julietta A., Natalie J. Bales, Sage A. Myers, et al. "The Hypothalamic-Pituitary-Adrenal Axis: Development, Programming Actions of Hormones, and Maternal-Fetal Interactions." *Frontiers in Behavioral Neuroscience* (January 13, 2021), 1–21.

Shires, Deirdre A., Daphna Stroumsa, Kim D. Jaffee et al., "Primary Care Clinicians' Willingness to Care for Transgender Patients," *The Annals of Family Medicine* 16, no. 6 (November 2018).

Sicherman, Barbara. "The Uses of a Diagnosis: Doctors, Patients, and Neurasthenia." *Journal of the History of Medicine and Allied Sciences* 32, no. 1 (January 1977), 33–54.

Siegel, Bernie S. *Love, Medicine and Miracles.* New York: HarperCollins, 1986.

Sigmund, Barbara Boggs. "I Didn't Give Myself Cancer." *The New York Times* (December 30, 1989), A25.

Silverstein, Arthur M. "Autoimmunity Versus Horror Autotoxicus: The Struggle for Recognition." *Nature Immunology* 2, no. 4 (May 2001), 279–81.

Singh Ospina, N., K. A. Phillips, R. Rodriguez-Gutierrez, et al. "Eliciting the Patient's Agenda—Secondary Analysis of Recorded Clinical Encounters." *Journal of General Internal Medicine* 34, (2019), 36–40.

Singh, S. K., and H. J. Girschick. "Lyme Borreliosis: From Infection to Autoimmunity." *Clinical Microbiology and Infection* 10, no. 7 (2004), 598–614.

Smatti, Maria K., Farhan S. Cyprian, Gheyath K. Nasralla, et al. "Viruses and Autoimmunity: A Review on the Potential Interaction and Molecular Mechanisms." *Viruses* 11, no. 8 (August 2019), 762.

Smith-Rosenberg, Carroll. "The Hysterical Woman: Sex Roles and Role Conflict in Nineteenth-Century America." *Social Research* 39, no. 4 (Winter 1972), 652–78.

Smith-Rosenberg, Carroll, and Charles Rosenberg. "The Female Animal: Medical and Biological Views of Woman and Her Role in Nineteenth-Century America." *The Journal of American History* 60, no. 2 (September 1973), 332–56.

Sonnenburg, Justin, and Erica Sonnenburg. *The Good Gut: Taking Control of Your Weight, Your Mood, and Your Long-Term Health.* New York: Penguin Books, 2015.

Sontag, Susan. *Alice in Bed: A Play.* New York: Farrar, Straus and Giroux, 1993.

———. *Conversations with Susan Sontag.* Edited by Leland Poague. Jackson: University Press of Mississippi, 1997.

———. *Illness as Metaphor and AIDS and Its Metaphors.* New York: Farrar, Straus and Giroux, 2003.

Specter, Michael. "Germs Are Us." *The New Yorker* (October 22, 2012), 32–39.

Spiegel, David, Helena C. Kraemer, Joan R. Bloom, and Ellen Gottheil. "Effect of Psychosocial Treatment on Survival of Patients with Metastatic Breast Cancer." *The Lancet* 334, no. 8668 (1989), 888–91.

Spiegel, David, Lisa D. Butler, Janine Giese-Davis, et al. "Effects of Supportive-Expressive Group Therapy on Survival of Patients with Metastatic Breast Cancer: A Randomized Prospective Trial." *Cancer* 110, no. 5 (September 2007), 1130–38.

Spreng, M. "Possible Health Effects of Noise Induced Cortisol Increase." *Noise Health* 2, no. 7 (2000), 59–64.

Starr, Paul. *The Social Transformation of American Medicine: The Rise of a Sovereign Profession and the Making of a Vast Industry.* New York: Basic Books, 2017.

Stauffer, Jill. *Ethical Loneliness: The Injustice of Not Being Heard.* New York: Columbia University Press, 2018.

Steinberg, M., E. D. Benjamin, et al. "Bacteria and the Neural Code." *The New England Journal of Medicine* 371 (2014), 2131–33.

Steptoe, Andrew, and Mika Kivimäki. "Stress and Cardiovascular Disease." *Nature Reviews Cardiology* 9, no. 6 (April 2012), 360-70.

Sternberg, Esther M. *Healing Spaces: The Science of Place and Well-Being.* Cambridge, MA: Belknap Press, 2009.

Stevens, Patricia E., and Pamela K. Pletsch. "Informed Consent and the History of Inclusion of Women in Clinical Research." *Health Care for Women International* 23 (2002), 809–19.

Stitt, Jennifer. "Will COVID-19 Strengthen Our Bonds?" *Guernica* (May 12, 2020), https://www.guernicamag.com/will-covid-19-strengthen-our-bonds/.

Stix, Gary. "A Malignant Flame." *Scientific American* (July 1, 2008), https://www.scientificamerican.com/article/a-malignant-flame-2008-07/.

Strachan, D. P. "Hay Fever, Hygiene, and Household Size." *British Medical Journal* 299, no. 6710 (November 18, 1989), 1259–60.

Strouse, Jean. *Alice James: A Biography.* With a preface by Colm Tóibín. New York: New York Review of Books Classics, 2011.

Stubbs, John. *John Donne: The Reformed Soul.* New York: W. W. Norton, 2008.

"Study: CDC's Two-Tier Lyme Testing Was Inaccurate in More Than 70% of Cases." *LymeDisease.org News* (February 26, 2020), https://www.lymedisease.org/study-cdcs-two-tier-lyme-testing-was-inaccurate-in-more-than-70-of-cases/.

Styron, William. *Darkness Visible: A Memoir of Madness*. New York: Vintage, 1992.

"Susan Sontag Found Crisis of Cancer Added a Fierce Intensity to Life." *The New York Times* (January 30, 1978), 19.

Sweet, Victoria. *Slow Medicine: The Way to Healing*. New York: Riverhead Books, 2017.

Talley, Colin Lee. "The Emergence of Multiple Sclerosis, 1870–1950: A Puzzle of Historical Epidemiology." *Perspectives in Biology and Medicine* 48, no. 3 (2005), 383–95.

Tate, Leslie. "Study Finds Evidence of Persistent Lyme Infection in Brain Despite Aggressive Antibiotic Therapy." *Tulane News* (May 17, 2021), https://news.tulane.edu/pr/study-finds-evidence-persistent-lyme-infection-brain-despite-aggressive-antibiotic-therapy.

Thernstrom, Melanie. *The Pain Chronicles: Cures, Myths, Mysteries, Prayers, Diaries, Brain Scans, Healing, and the Science of Suffering*. New York: Farrar, Straus and Giroux, 2010.

Tick-Borne Disease Working Group. *2018 Report to Congress*. Washington, DC: U.S. Department of Health and Human Services (2018), https://www.hhs.gov/sites/default/files/tbdwg-report-to-congress-2018.pdf.

Tillisch, Kirsten, Jennifer Labus, Lisa Kilpatrick, et al. "Consumption of Fermented Milk Product with Probiotic Modulates Brain Activity." *Gastroenterology* 144, no. 7 (June 2013), 1394–401.

Todd, K. H., C. Deaton, A. P. D'Adamo, and L. Goe. "Ethnicity and Analgesic Practice." *Annals of Emergency Medicine* 35, no. 1 (January 2000), 11–16.

van Nood, Els, Anne Vrieze, Max Nieuwdorp, et al. "Duodenal Infusion of Donor Feces for Recurrent *Clostridium difficile*." *The New England Journal of Medicine* 368 (January 31, 2013), 407–15.

Velasquez-Manoff, Moises. *An Epidemic of Absence: A New Way of Understanding Allergies and Autoimmune Diseases*. New York: Scribner, 2012.

Vidali, Amy. "Hysterical Again: The Gastrointestinal Woman in Medical Discourse." *Journal of Medical Humanities* 34 (2013), 33–57.

Von Hertzen, L. C., and T. Haahtela. "Asthma and Atopy—the Price of Affluence?" *Allergy* 59, no. 2 (February 2004), 124–37.

Wahls, Terry, with Eve Adamson. *The Wahls Protocol: A Radical New Way to Treat All Chronic Autoimmune Conditions Using Paleo Principles*. New York: Avery, 2014.

Wailoo, Keith. *Pain: A Political History*. Baltimore: Johns Hopkins University Press, 2014.

Wang, Aolin, Dimitri Panagopoulos Abrahamsson, Ting Jiang, et al. "Suspect Screening, Prioritization, and Confirmation of Environmental Chemicals in Maternal-Newborn Pairs from San Francisco." *Environmental Science and Technology* 55, no. 8 (2021), 5037–49.

Washington, Harriet A. *Infectious Madness: The Surprising Science of How We "Catch" Mental Illness*. New York: Little, Brown, 2015.

Williamson, A. M., and Anne-Marie Feyer. "Moderate Sleep Deprivation Produces Impairments in Cognitive and Motor Performance Equivalent to Legally Prescribed Levels of Alcohol Intoxication." *Occupational and Environmental Medicine* 57, no. 10 (October 2000), 649–55.

Williamson, John B., Eric C. Porges, Damon G. Lamb, and Stephen W. Porges. "Maladaptive Autonomic Regulation in PTSD Accelerates Physiological Aging." *Frontiers in Psychology* 5 (January 2015), 1571.

Wilson, James L. *Adrenal Fatigue: The 21st Century Stress Syndrome*. With a foreword by Jonathan V. Wright. Smart Publications, 2002.

Wiman, Christian. *He Held Radical Light: The Art of Faith, the Faith of Art*. New York: Farrar, Straus and Giroux, 2018.

Woolf, Steven H., Laudan Aron, Lisa Dubay, et al. "How Are Income and Wealth Linked to Health and Longevity?" Urban Institute, Center on Society and Health (April 2015), https://www.urban.org/sites/default/files/publication/49116/2000178 -How-are-Income-and-Wealth-Linked-to-Health-and-Longevity.pdf.

Woolf, Virginia. *On Being Ill*. Ashfield, MA: Paris Press, 2002.

World Health Organization Regional Office for Europe. "Lyme Borreliosis in Europe." European Centre for Disease Prevention and Control (2014), https://www.ecdc .europa.eu/sites/portal/files/media/en/healthtopics/vectors/world-health-day-2014 /Documents/factsheet-lyme-borreliosis.pdf.

Wormser, Gary P., Raymond J. Dattwyler, Eugene D. Shapiro, et al. "The Clinical Assessment, Treatment, and Prevention of Lyme Disease, Human Granulocytic Anaplasmosis, and Babesiosis: Clinical Practice Guidelines by the Infectious Diseases Society of America." *Clinical Infectious Diseases* 43, no. 9 (November 2006), 1089–134.

Wormser G. P., D. McKenna, C. Scavarda, et al. "Co-infections in Persons with Early Lyme Disease, New York, USA." *Emerging Infectious Diseases* 25, no. 4 (2019), 748–52.

Wybran, J. "Enkephalins and Endorphins as Modifiers of the Immune System: Present and Future." *Federation Proceedings* 44, no. 1 (January 1985), 92–94.

Xu, Huihui, Meijie Lui, Jinfeng Cao, et al. "The Dynamic Interplay Between the Gut Microbiota and Autoimmune Diseases." *Journal of Immunology Research* (2019).

Yang, Chen-Yen, Patrick S. C. Leung, Iannis E. Adamopoulos, and M. Eric Gershwin. "The Implication of Vitamin D and Autoimmunity: A Comprehensive Review." *Clinical Review of Allergy Immunology* 45, no. 2 (October 2013), 217–26.

Young, Jarred, Luke Parkitny, and David McLain. "The Use of Low-Dose Naltrexone (LDN) as a Novel Anti-Inflammatory Treatment for Chronic Pain." *Clinical Rheumatology* 33, no. 4 (2014), 451–59.

Zhang, Zimu, and Rongxin Zhang. "Epigenetics in Autoimmune Diseases: Pathogenesis and Prospects for Therapy." *Autoimmunity Reviews* 14, no. 10 (2015), 854–63.

Zuo, Y., et al. *Science Translational Medicine* 12, no. 570 (November 18, 2020).

Index